Advance Praise for
Words of Wisdom From
Pivotal Nurse Leaders

"Be prepared for an exhilarating read! Beth Houser and Kathy Player take you inside the thinking of nurse leaders who have paved the way for the profession of nursing. The authors have created a beautifully written volume that provides guidance and wisdom to those interested in nursing leadership. In strong, compelling voices, the authors explore key topics. The use of quotes and reflections, as well as the magnificent photographs, makes this a must read. This book should inspire all who read it."

Jeanette Ives Frickson, RN, MS, FAAN
Senior Vice President for Patient Care Services
Chief Nurse Executive
Massachusetts General Hospital

"This is a stunning addition to the nursing leadership literature. The words and experiences of some of our most esteemed leaders provide much needed reflection in our busy lives. I especially appreciate the pairing of the photographs with the insights. It is a book that will bring both pleasure and wisdom to the reader."

Pamela Thompson MS, RN, FAAN
Chief Executive Officer
American Organization of Nurse Executives (AONE)

D1605552

"This is an inspiring volume filled with words from leaders in nursing. These words reflect more than their experiences—they reveal the imagery that inspires them in their work, advice about responding to inevitable errors and continuing on, and self-awareness of their own humanness. Some of the advice is particularly useful, such as finding someone with the skill set that complements your own, shaping the message and language to your audience, and persevering through tough times. This little collection belongs on your desk, not the coffee table!"

Nancy Fugate Woods, PhD, RN, FAAN
The Robert G. and Jean A. Reid Endowed Dean in Nursing
Professor, Family and Child Nursing
University of Washington School of Nursing, Seattle

WORDS OF WISDOM

from Pivotal Nurse Leaders

BETH P. HOUSER, DNSC, FNP, NEA-BC

KATHY N. PLAYER, EDD, RN, MS-N, MBA

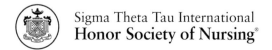

Sigma Theta Tau International
Honor Society of Nursing®

SIGMA THETA TAU INTERNATIONAL
Editor-in-Chief: Jeff Burnham
Acquisitions Editor: Cynthia Saver, RN, MS
Development Editor: Carla Hall
Copy Editors: Linda Puffer & Jane Palmer
Photo Editor: Jane Palmer
Researcher: Paula Jeffers

Cover Design, Interior Design and Page Composition by: Rebecca Harmon

Printed in the United States of America
Printing and Binding by Printing Partners   PARTNERS

Sigma Theta Tau International
550 West North Street
Indianapolis, IN 46202
Visit our Web site at **www.nursingknowledge.org/STTI/books** for more information on our books.

ISBN-10: 1-930538-83-9
ISBN-13: 978-1-930538-83-2

Library of Congress Cataloging-in-Publication Data

Houser, Beth, 1957-
  Words of wisdom from pivotal nurse leaders / Beth P. Houser and Kathy N. Player.
     p. ; cm.
  Includes bibliographical references.
  ISBN 978-1-930538-83-2
  1. Nurses--Supervision of. 2. Nursing services--Administration. 3. Leadership. I. Player, Kathy,
1962- II. Sigma Theta Tau International. III. Title.
  [DNLM: 1. Nursing, Supervisory--organization & administration--United States. 2. Leadership--
United States. 3. Nurses--United States. WY 105 H842w 2008]
  RT86.45.H68 2008
  362.17'3--dc22
                                        2008029545
  First Printing
  2008

DEDICATION

Let whoever is in charge keep this simple question in her head (*not,* how can I always do this right thing myself, but) how can I provide for this right thing to always be done?

—Nightingale, F. (1859). *Notes on nursing: What it is and What it is Not.* London: Harrison & Sons. (p. 24).

We dedicate this book to the 23 amazing nurse leaders who provided their biographical stories published in *Pivotal Moments in Nursing: Leaders Who Changed the Path of a Profession*, volumes I and II. The wisdom, philosophies, teachings, and life-long learning each of these leaders convey helps showcase how nurse leaders can "provide for this right thing to always be done" for patients and health care providers.

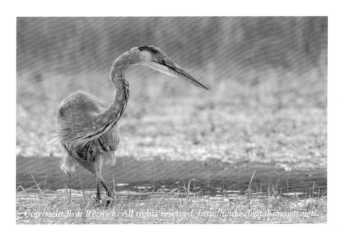

Acknowledgements

We would like to thank the Robert Wood Johnson (RWJ) Foundation for the continued commitment to building health care leaders. The RWJ Executive Nurse Fellows Program has been an inspiration and pathway for us to collaborate with the remarkable leaders who became the focus of our books. We expect many RWJ Executive Nurse Fellows will one day have their leadership stories told by future authors as they are making today's health care history.

Thanks to my remarkable friend and highly competent administrative assistant, Cathy Collette, for helping me collect and organize potential contributions for this book. Cathy is one of those remarkable people who quietly and efficiently move mountains. And, with great appreciation, I thank my family for their support, patience, and inspiration. My children—Jessica, Adam, Rob, and Kevin—have filled my life with joy and pride. Each one of you has so much to offer, and I am confident that you will live your dreams. I thank you for the laughter, love, and caring. Thanks to Bill and Sandy who have been more than siblings—you have been my sounding board and vision when I could not see. You have enriched my life with your remarkable families and a lifetime of hilarious memories.

—Beth

Thanks once again to Grand Canyon University under the leadership of Executive Chairman Brent Richardson. You have provided me the support to continuously give back to the nursing profession while learning under your tutelage. The turnaround story of Grand Canyon University is nothing short of its own leadership story worth publishing someday soon! And, I would like to thank my husband, parents, and dear friends Michael and Arlene. You are the cheering section in my sometimes chaotic-paced life.

—Kathy

ABOUT THE AUTHORS

BETH P. HOUSER, DNSc, FNP, NEA-BC

Dr. Beth Houser is Chief Nursing Officer of Baylor Regional Medical Center at Grapevine in Texas. Previous leadership roles include Director of Critical Care and Telemetry at Scottsdale Healthcare (2005-2008) and Director of Nursing Research and the Magnet Project for John C. Lincoln-North Mountain (2002-2005) in Arizona. Beth has been a Magnet appraiser for the American Nurses Credentialing Center since 2002 and has been involved in all aspects of the application process and program evolution. She is a Robert Wood Johnson Executive Nurse Fellow (2002 cohort). She holds a BSN, an MSN as a family nurse practitioner, and a doctorate from Johns Hopkins University School of Nursing where her study was devoted to educating nurse scientists to use large databases to answer global health care questions. She guest lectures, presents Magnet information at national conferences, and publishes on both leadership and Magnet topics. She has three children: Jessica, the mother of two beautiful children; Rob, a Lance Corporal in the United States Marine Corps currently serving a tour of duty in Iraq; and Kevin, a student at the University of Arizona.

KATHY N. PLAYER, EdD, RN, MS-N, MBA

Dr. Kathy Player is President of Grand Canyon University. She previously held the positions of Provost and Chief Academic Officer, Grand Canyon University, and Dean of the Ken Blanchard College of Business and the College of Entrepreneurship, Chair of Professional Studies, and Director for the RN-BSN program. Kathy coordinated the development of an HLC-accredited Master of Science in Leadership program that has been widely received by the health care community. She is a Robert Wood Johnson Executive Nurse Fellow (2002 cohort). Kathy has a global interest in improving the nursing profession and health care by providing nurses access to business, management, and leadership education. She lobbies actively at both local and national levels on behalf of nurses and nursing issues. Kathy has worked with Thai baccalaureate nursing students and faculty in Trang, Thailand, participated in a health care leadership exchange in Cuba, and participated in two different Global Nursing Exchange trips to Mexico. She has worked on many successful health care proposition campaigns within Arizona, and she successfully coordinated efforts to receive a Leadership Initiative grant and a statewide Nursing Workforce Environment grant through the Arizona Nurses Association. She holds a BSN, a master's in counseling, a master's in nursing, a doctorate, and an MBA.

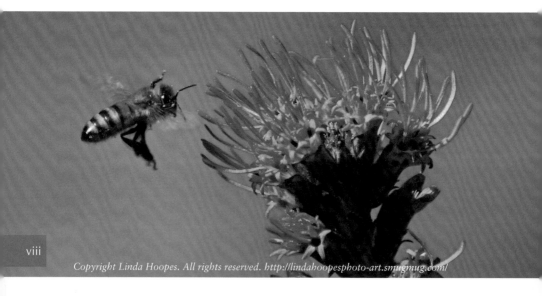

TABLE OF CONTENTS

FOREWORD

Being a nurse leader implies both privilege and responsibility; the privilege comes in having the opportunity to make a difference in so many people's lives; the responsibility comes in ensuring that you are traveling on the right path since the choices you make impact followers, both directly and indirectly. Making the right choices and positively impacting lives requires a high degree of wisdom; a trait clearly in abundance in the contributors to this book.

Wisdom is defined by the Free Dictionary as insight or the ability to discern or judge what is true, right, or lasting. WorldNet's definition is similar in that it suggests wisdom represents accumulated knowledge or erudition or enlightenment as well as the ability to apply knowledge or experience with common sense and insight.

The problem with wisdom is that being wise does not automatically translate to the ability to successfully share that wisdom with others. That's where leadership comes in. Leaders are those individuals who are out front, moving forward, taking risks, and challenging the status quo to make a difference in the lives of their followers. Leaders recognize the importance and absolute necessity of sharing their wisdom as part of the socialization, mentoring, and career development of others.

In *Words of Wisdom from Pivotal Nurse Leaders*, Beth Houser and Kathy Player share the wisdom acquired by some of the nursing profession's greatest leaders. Some of the wisdom is shared in the form of stories and lessons learned from difficult life experiences. Other wisdom comes from education and reflects an understanding gained only through an immersion in the science of the profession. Other wisdom comes in the form of intuition, feelings, or reflections based upon a lifetime dedicated to working with and for others.

All of the contributors to this book are thought leaders in the profession; those individuals who are recognized among their peers for innovative ideas and who demonstrate the confidence to promote those ideas. All of the contributions reflect emotional intelligence—a self awareness about one's values, beliefs, and the ability to perceive, identify, manage, and integrate emotions in connecting with other individuals.

The wisdom shared in this book is applicable to nurses in all career stages. Indeed, the wisdom shared in this book transcends professional application and simply focuses on the potential we all have to be leaders and to make a difference. The need for courage, risk taking, action, commitment, vision, passion, integrity, self-awareness, communication, flexibility, humility, and diplomacy emerge. Loss, rejection, and frustration are revealed as potential costs of our leadership journeys. But the final message in this legacy of shared wisdom is that we all have the ability to make a difference

Carol J. Huston, MSN, DPA, FAAN
2007-2009 President
Honor Society of Nursing, Sigma Theta Tau International

Contributing Authors

Faye Glenn Abdellah, RN, EdD, ScD, FAAN

Faye Glenn Abdellah is recognized internationally for her public service in nursing, education, and health care. She was the chief nurse officer and deputy surgeon general with the U.S. Public Health Service, where she retired with the rank of rear admiral, and was the first nurse to hold the title of deputy surgeon general for the United States.

Linda Aiken, RN, PhD, FAAN, FRCN

Linda Aiken is director of the Center for Health Outcomes and Policy Research, the Claire M. Fagin Leadership Professor of Nursing, a professor of sociology, and a senior fellow at the Leonard Davis Institute for Health Economics at the University of Pennsylvania. Aiken co-directs the National Council on Physician and Nurse Supply, addressing national and global shortages of health professionals.

Richard Henry Carmona, RN, MD, MPH, FACS

Richard Henry Carmona served as a special forces medic for the U.S. Army during the Vietnam War where he earned distinction for bravery and valor in combat. He went on to become a nurse and then a physician-surgeon, eventually becoming the 17th surgeon general of the United States. He is president of the nonprofit Canyon Ranch Institute in Arizona and recipient of the first distinguished professorship in public health at the University of Arizona's Mel and Enid Zuckerman College of Public Health.

M. Elizabeth Carnegie, RN, DPA, FAAN

M. Elizabeth Carnegie was a ground-breaking nurse and educator who championed the cause of African-American nurses. Carnegie initiated the baccalaureate nursing program at the historically Black Hampton University in Virginia and she served as dean and professor of the School of Nursing at Florida A & M University. A prolific author, Carnegie served as an editor for the American Journal of Nursing Company from 1953-1978. Editor emerita of *Nursing Research*, Carnegie died in 2008.

Shirley Sears Chater, RN, PhD, FAAN

Shirley Sears Chater served in the role of commissioner of the United States Social Security Administration from 1993 until 1997. Prior to that, she was the president of Texas Woman's University from 1986-1993. She sits on several boards and lectures on public policy and on economic and social issues concerning the aging population in the United States.

Luther Christman, RN, PhD, FAAN

Luther Christman is recognized internationally as a leader, innovator, and consultant to nursing schools, health care agencies, and professional organizations in nursing and medicine. He has consulted nationally to more than 14 countries in the area of nursing education and health care.

Joyce C. Clifford, RN, PhD, FAAN

Joyce C. Clifford is president and CEO of The Institute for Nursing Healthcare Leadership (INHL). Before founding INHL, she served as senior vice president and nurse-in-chief at Beth Israel Deaconess Medical Center in Boston, Massachusetts, USA, for more than 25 years. Clifford is an established author and consultant on the subject of organizational restructuring and the development of a professional practice model.

Leah Curtin, RN, MS, MA, FAAN

Leah Curtin is a clinical professor of nursing at the University of Cincinnati College of Nursing and Health and was editor in chief of *Nursing Management* for 20 years. She is best known for her advocacy role in ethics in health care.

Rheba de Tornyay, EdD, FAAN

Rheba de Tornyay is Professor Emeritus and a former dean of the School of Nursing, University of Washington. Her longstanding commitments to excellence in nursing education and the role of nursing in health policy led to the establishment of the annual Rheba de Tornyay award for excellence in undergraduate teaching and the de Tornyay Center on Healthy Aging.

Sue Karen Donaldson, RN, PhD, FAAN

Sue Karen Donaldson, former dean of the Johns Hopkins University School of Nursing, is a pioneer in the development of nursing research and is known internationally for her basic science research in cellular skeletal and cardiac muscle physiology.

Claire Fagin, RN, PhD, FAAN

Claire Fagin, the first woman to serve as president of an Ivy League university when she served as interim president of the University of Pennsylvania, has blended an interest in consumer health issues with professional health and nursing issues. She is a consultant to foundations, national programs, and educational institutions.

Vernice D. Ferguson, RN, MA, FAAN, FRCN

Vernice Ferguson, a longstanding advocate for gender and ethnic parity in health care, spent more than 20 years as a top nurse executive in United States federal service, including 12 years as the nurse leader for the Department of Veterans Affairs, the largest organized nursing service in the world with more than 60,000 nurses.

Loretta C. Ford, EdD, FAAN

Loretta C. Ford is recognized as the founder of the nurse practitioner movement. She has served as dean of the School of Nursing at the University of Rochester and Director of Nursing at the University Medical Center. She has devoted her career to practice, education, consultation and influencing health services inquiry. She is currently Professor and Program Director for the Commonwealth Fund's Executive Nurse Leadership Program.

Ada Sue Hinshaw, RN, PhD, FAAN

Ada Sue Hinshaw was the first permanent director of the National Institute of Nursing Research at the National Institutes of Health. She is a professor and former dean of the University of Michigan's School of Nursing and is internationally recognized as a contributor to nursing research. She is the dean of the Graduate School of Nursing at The Uniformed Services University of the Health Sciences in Bethesda, Maryland.

Ruth Watson Lubic, CNM, EdD, FAAN, FACNM

Ruth Watson Lubic, a tireless fighter for families and midwifery care, was the first nurse to be awarded the prestigious MacArthur (genius) Fellowship in 1993. Her vision ultimately led to the establishment of the first freestanding child-bearing center in the United States—the Developing Families Center in Washington, D.C.—supporting one of the most underserved populations in the United States.

Margaret L. McClure, RN, EdD, FAAN

Margaret L. McClure took a question and turned it around. Instead of "why do nurses leave?" she asked "why do nurses stay?" The result is what is known worldwide as "Magnet." For almost 20 years she was the chief nursing officer at NYU Medical Center where she also served as the chief operating officer and hospital administrator.

Marla E. Salmon, RN, ScD, FAAN

Marla Salmon works on health care issues throughout the world. She is the Robert G. and Jean A. Reid Endowed Dean in Nursing and Professor, Family and Child Nursing, University of Washington School of Nursing, Seattle, Washington, USA. Most recently, Marla was dean and professor of the Nell Hodgson Woodruff School of Nursing, Emory University, Atlanta, Georgia, USA, and director of Emory University's Lillian Carter Center for International Nursing.

Judith Shamian, RN, PhD, LLD

Judith Shamian is president and CEO of VON Canada (Victorian Order of Nurses for Canada). Her youth was shaped by the circumstances that found her surviving three wars by the age of 23. Shamian serves on numerous national and international committees concerned with health services and systems knowledge, policy development, and nursing.

GRAYCE SILLS, RN, PhD, FAAN

Grayce Sills is professor emeritus at The Ohio State University College of Nursing. She is an internationally recognized scholar and a gifted, inspirational, and compassionate pioneer in the field of psychiatric mental health nursing.

KIRSTEN STALLKNECHT, RN, FAAN

Kirsten Stallknecht served 28 years as president of the Danish Nurses Organization and served several years as president of the International Council of Nurses. She has been involved with nursing both nationally and internationally.

MARGRETTA MADDEN STYLES, RN, EdD, FAAN

Margretta Madden Styles was recognized internationally for her contributions in academic nursing, credentialing, and professional organizations. Styles was recognized worldwide for her special expertise in professional issues, particularly regulation and credentialing. She died in 2005.

FLORENCE SCHORSKE WALD, RN, MN, MS, FAAN

Florence Schorske Wald was a pioneer of the hospice movement in the United States. Recognizing that the terminally ill have unique needs, she developed a hospice model that provides holistic and humanistic care for the dying person.

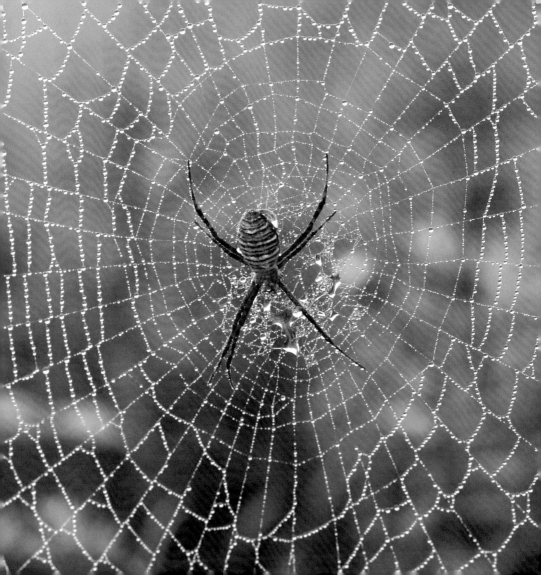

Tools in the Toolbox

Conventional wisdom has long held that leaders are born and not developed. That, however, seldom proves to be the case with nursing, where leadership is more often than not learned on the job. This section, "Tools in the Toolbox," provides an assortment of leadership tips from some of the profession's most exceptional leaders, offering nurses "lessons learned" tools for developing their own leadership styles and leading their organizations at a higher level.

"Tools in the Toolbox" is filled with helpful leadership wisdom for the myriad situations that nurses face every day. These tips provide insights on how to recover from mistakes, achieve success, temper and reframe a strong attitude, build teams, network, and develop diplomacy. As nurses, we are almost always drawn into the profession to care for and advocate on behalf of our patients. However, if we are not properly equipped, the day-to-day issues outside of patient care can become daunting and tax our ability to remain focused on the salient issues.

As a leader, you can decide which leadership tips best fit your needs and add them to your repertoire. Then you can adapt them to the particular situation you are managing. We hope you will find new tools to help you develop into the leader you were meant to be.

KNOWLEDGE IS POWER

—Linda Aiken

"Nurses don't read. You have to read and you have to have some way to communicate what the important issues are in the profession. By not reading, nurses don't realize that every other nurse is facing the same practice concerns, so they do not see the commonalities across different examples that would empower them. Instead, they reproduce things over and over and over again without realizing someone else has probably already done it, and they could build on that work in a more productive rather than redundant way."

Take the time to read the literature and gain direction from the great work of others.

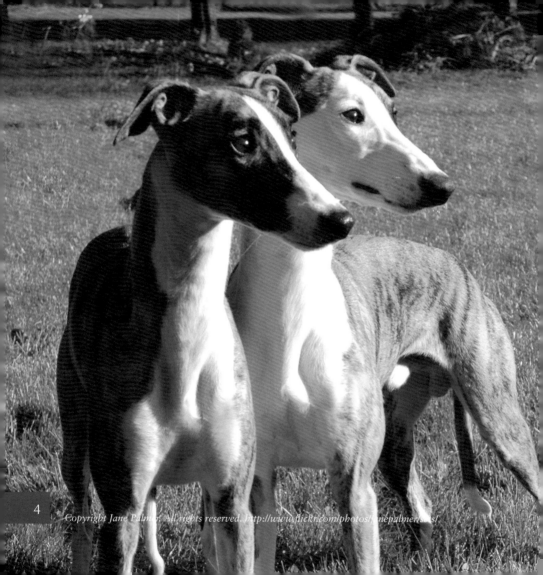

CHOOSING EXCELLENCE

—Vernice Ferguson

As a visionary seeking to advance nursing, Vernice kept her eye on "tomorrow" throughout her career. Excellence and enthusiasm have always been her secrets to success.

"You have to be enthusiastic and passionate about what you do and, of course, excellent at what you do and what you believe so it gets translated to other people."

Vernice never settled for mediocrity and knew excellence in her work would speak for itself. It is human nature to compare ourselves to others around us. One leadership lesson she learned early on is not to expend energy worrying about who has power or resources that you don't have. This form of unproductive competition leads to many hours a day, week, or month wasted in trivial, back-and-forth discussions among colleagues.

As Vernice models: Keep your nose down, work hard, and produce excellent results. Outcomes will speak for themselves, and everything else will follow.

DEFINING SUCCESS

—*Marla Salmon*

"Being strategic is extremely important, so that when you go into a situation, you know in advance what you consider to be a success. Once you are involved, the stakes escalate and you become an unfair judge of whether or not it was successful; this is particularly important when working with people you don't necessarily like."

Being strategic allows you to focus on the why of a position, project, or initiative. One example of this is when an organization decides to pursue Magnet or Baldridge recognition. The original marker of success is commonly defined as creating an environment of excellence. The why enculturates systems of performance excellence for superior patient, staff, and organizational outcomes. The stakes begin to escalate when the program review nears and the definition of success morphs into a quest for trophy-type recognition. The original goal of creating an environment of excellence can be overshadowed by the desire to publicly proclaim the victory. Many good organizations have given up on a great process because of perceived failure to win the trophy. The original success marker of creating

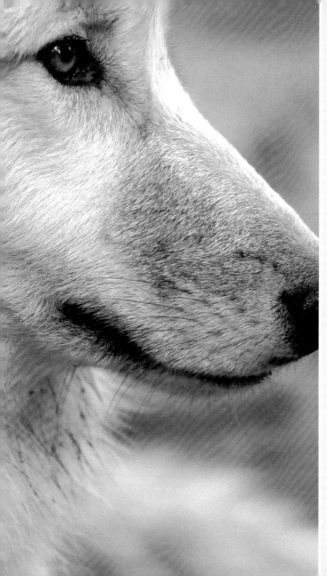

an infrastructure of superior outcomes gets lost in the emotion of being told the organization fell short—when, in fact, remarkable progress may have been made. Leaders must learn to embrace critique as a gift from experts and grow stronger from it.

Being a Change Agent

—Faye Abdellah

Effecting change can be easier than it appears. Faye Abdellah reflects upon how important "finding the hook" can be in making change. The leader must figure out why change is of value to the currently existing conditions. What must the leader understand about the current situation and the anticipated outcomes if he or she is to successfully effect change within an organization?

When making a public presentation to a group, the speaker must ask: Who is my audience, and what do they hope to get out of this? When a leader attempts to make change, it is important to understand which aspects of the change appeal to others. How are you going to sell the vision?

MEASURING SUCCESS IN SMALL INCREMENTS

—Kirsten Stallknecht

Celebrating successes in small increments is important, especially when the journey to the finish line is long. This helps to maintain morale and keep the focus on the ultimate goal. Kirsten made the mistake that most leaders make when stepping into a new position of authority and power.

"I wanted to change everything at one time. It was like having a full plate of food and not knowing quite how to use a knife and fork."

Kirsten learned to measure success in small increments or steps. The path of reaching her goal was more important than the speed of getting to the finish line. Her nursing skills of prioritization were critical to making positive changes in incremental steps. She could not turn around an organization's weak finances overnight, but she could turn them around—and she did—over time.

BUILDING A CHAMPIONSHIP TEAM

—Shirley Chater

"Radical change cannot occur without ownership and buy-in from employees," as Shirley Chater realized upon accepting her position as the new president of Texas Woman's University. Faced with a crisis situation when the commission of higher education wanted to merge Texas Woman's University with the University of North Texas, Shirley organized a vision, mission, and set of objectives to guide the organization into the future, while still ensuring support from the employees.

Leaders do not work alone. Instead, they act as one with their team of employees. Strive to become a championship team instead of a team made up of individual champions.

Think of a time when you successfully built a team; reflect upon how you did it and why you chose key individuals.

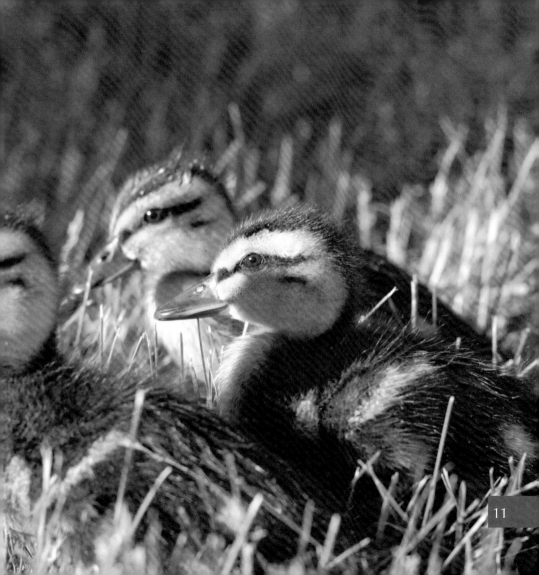

DIPLOMACY

—Faye Abdellah

Some great leaders learn quickly from their earlier lessons, while others have a fierce sense of determination to effect change without regard for the consequences. This was true of Faye Abdellah, who readily admits she might have been a slow learner when it came to using diplomacy to accomplish her goals. She learned her life lessons through the "school of hard knocks," so to speak.

Upon receiving her first faculty teaching position, Faye wanted to update the nursing textbook her students were using. The dean would not support this change. Faye asked all her students to gather in the school courtyard and bring their course textbooks. Before long, she had a bonfire going and tossed all the outdated books into the blaze! This reactive, intensely passionate response did not move her agenda. What it did was get her fired. It took 25-30 years for her to become the skilled diplomat who rose to the level of deputy surgeon general under C. Everett Koop.

Reflect on your style for dealing with potentially reactive situations. Try to cultivate the diplomat in yourself.

LEARNING FROM OTHERS' MISTAKES

—Grayce Sills

Some of the best lessons learned along the path of life are those included in the category of *what not to do to another human being*. Grayce had one instructor in school who developed negative student nicknames. In Grayce's case, her nickname was "dumb bunny." Worse yet, Grayce came to believe she was, as her instructor referenced, a dumb bunny. Years later, with much more wisdom, experience, and confidence under her belt, she could look back and understand that negative and carelessly used words can be damaging, especially if they cause people to question their own aptitude and intelligence. This painful lesson taught Grayce never to be sarcastic or cynical when providing feedback to students. This experience made her a stronger, more sensitive teacher precisely because she learned, from her own painful feelings of self-doubt, what not to do to someone else.

Have you ever received feedback that did more damage than good at the time? How long did it take you to process those words into something that provided helpful feedback?

CRUCIAL CONVERSATIONS

—Shirley Chater

Shirley learned early in her career that all leaders will have crucial conversations with employees who might not be the right fit for their position. One of her early mentors taught her that you should reinforce the positives and strengths of the person at the same time you let the person know it is time for a change in that particular department. The employee can then walk away feeling as though he or she has just been given a distinct honor, rather than demoted or terminated.

Leaving someone "whole" during a crucial conversation, while getting a difficult point across, is a skillful art in interpersonal communications. The focus remains on the individual and not the task. Practice this skill with a mentor or other supportive individual in your life.

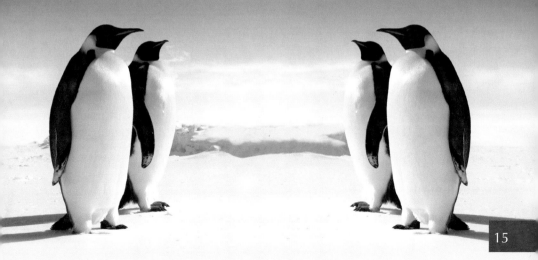

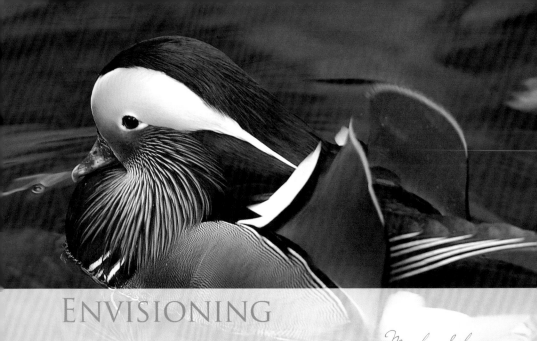

ENVISIONING

—Marla Salmon

Marla believes that everyone has a "coloring book." Formulated in our early years, it creates the outlines of who we will become. Sometimes we color our life possibilities inside the lines and other times outside the lines, but these possibilities occur because "at one point we created space in our imagination for this to be." Marla calls *vision* the coloring book for an organization.

16

MOVING THE AGENDA BY BUILDING RELATIONSHIPS

—Ruth Lubic

Making an impact in the nursing profession through the advancement of midwifery was no easy task for Ruth Lubic. "It is important to realize that you will require a lot of help from a lot of people when advancing a forward-looking agenda. You can't afford to make enemies, and confrontation doesn't help much. There is no way around it for a successful leader: You either navigate and play politics, or lose."

Ruth could have faced off against her colleagues in medicine to "fight the good fight" for bringing midwifery to the forefront of nursing. However, she knew that would be taking the long and winding road. It was easier—and wiser—to take her medical colleagues under her wing and circumnavigate issues before they arose. While it was not an easy journey for Ruth, in the end her medical colleagues greatly respected her fortitude, passion, and knowledge. She became the first nurse to receive the prestigious MacArthur "genius" Fellowship grant in 1993.

NETWORKING

—Judith Shamian

A strong leader has a powerful network of colleagues. "If properly net-worked, one should only be a few degrees of separation from the col-league who has the solution."

Interestingly enough, the higher up one goes on the career ladder with title, salary, and benefits, the more difficult it is to quickly change jobs when necessary. Executive vice president positions are not always open when and where they are needed. In an ever-changing health care en-vironment, a network is critical. Leaders and leaders-to-be should be so well-networked that they can replace their current job for equal or greater pay in three phone calls or less. This concept stresses the importance of being networked among colleagues of equal or higher stature through professional associations and fellowships, so that you are known for your work ethic and accomplishments.

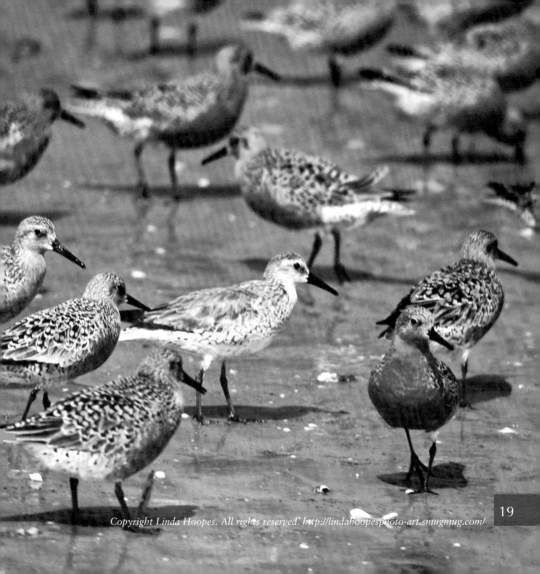

19

Role Modeling

—Marla Salmon

Marla's most admired leadership qualities include:

- "Never forget to leave the campground cleaner than you found it;
- Match potential with opportunity; and
- Apply the vision of what *is* possible and what *can make it* possible."

Celebrating

—Marla Salmon

"Celebrate your successes, keep a sense of humor, and stay in touch with younger people."

For a leader, initiatives of great magnitude require extensive planning and collaboration. When the goal is finally achieved, the celebration is forgotten as you move onto another project. This is a missed opportunity to say thank you and gather momentum for the next hurdle. Marla believes that humor brings everyone to the same level and eases the tension. Staying in touch with younger people keeps you—and your leadership—contemporary and energized.

Knowing When It Is Time to Leave

—Judith Shamian

"Knowing when the time has come to leave an organization is something every leader should know. As important as it is to work through changes, it is equally as important to know when to get off the bus."

Believe it or not, this can be one of the most difficult lessons to learn when leaders are personally invested in their organizations. Judith applied for a vice president of nursing position and was passed over for a woman recruited from outside the organization. The candidate had a very different leadership style, which Judith realized would clash with her own. She knew that the combination would not work for the long term—it was time to seek employment elsewhere.

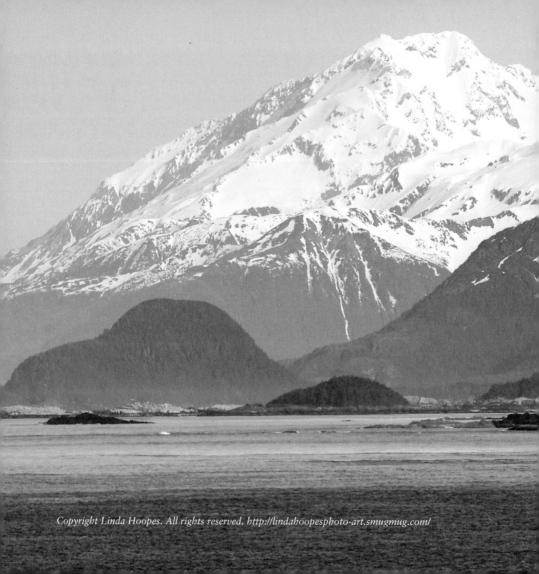

2

Leadership Courage

With leadership comes the risk of failure. Courage is an essential element of good leadership, yet it is interesting to note that strong leaders often face risky decisions on a daily basis and do not recognize their leadership as courageous. Leaders look at challenges as opportunities and will not stop until they have found sustainable solutions. The stakes may appear high and the stress excessive to aspiring leaders; however, the leader in the midst of the situation appears to thrive in response to the privilege of leading. The leader sets the emotional tone of calm and constructive direction in times of disaster and chaos. This is not as easy as great leaders make it appear. These gifted leaders are wise, strategic and resourceful. Some play off their courage, self-deprecatingly, and say they were not smart enough to fully know what they were up against. Don't believe them! Leaders have a vision of what should be and a roadmap on how to get there. Very few achieve success by luck.

Leadership courage illustrates the importance of challenging yourself throughout your nursing career—to push for what you deserve, to take the high road, and to come back stronger after rejection. Courage is the blood that runs through a leader's veins. It is essential for getting the job done. The leadership courage you desire to develop is wisely revealed in the following lessons from pivotal nurse leaders. Read on for insight into how you can become the courageous leader you want to be.

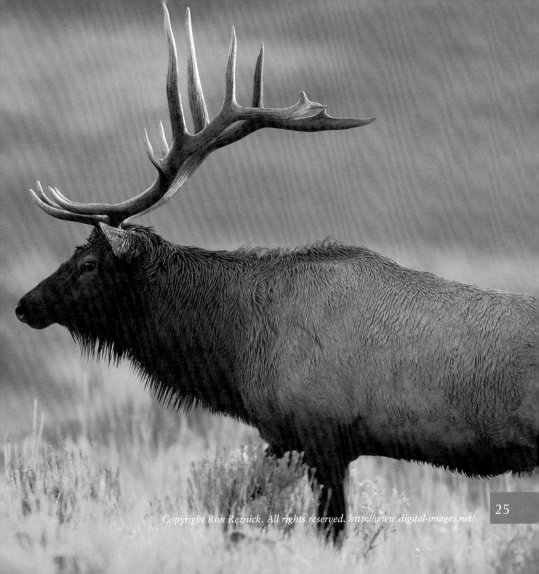

25

STEP OUT OF THE COMFORT ZONE

—Shirley Chater

Shirley would likely still be at Texas Woman's University if she had not been called to interview in Washington, DC, for the U.S. governmental position of head of the Social Security Administration (SSA). Shirley was a nurse with no in-depth knowledge of the SSA. What the president's administration was seeking was proven leadership, and *that* she had amply developed. Shirley demonstrated tremendous courage by stepping into a role that in many ways was foreign to her work history.

During her tenure as commissioner of the SSA, Shirley became aware of a client who asked to have his Social Security number changed because of the supposedly demonic connotations of the numbers "666" in sequence. Shirley's staff was adamant that this was against policy and could not be done. Shirley asked why a new number couldn't be issued. After hearing

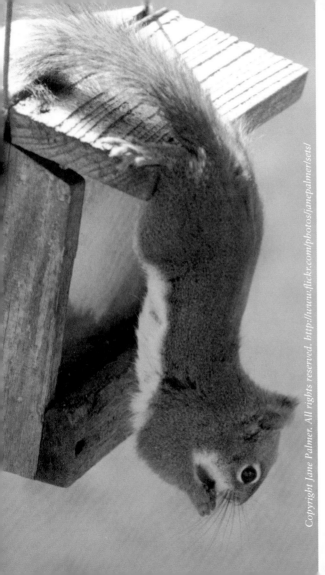

input from team members, it was decided that a new number could be issued. The customer's satisfaction was put before policy.

Leadership is about stretching oneself professionally and making those uncomfortable areas more comfortable. Seek experiences outside your comfort zone, and watch yourself ultimately master the challenge.

Simple Instructions

—Vernice Ferguson

"Be appropriate! Be bold! Be courageous!"

When Naiveté Works

—Kirsten Stallknecht

"Being naïve is a good thing at times of great risk." One tends to stand up unknowingly in the face of risk, without realizing the full commitment required by leadership in a situation until shortly after the "boat leaves the dock and starts taking on water." Then you will see a leader's true colors.

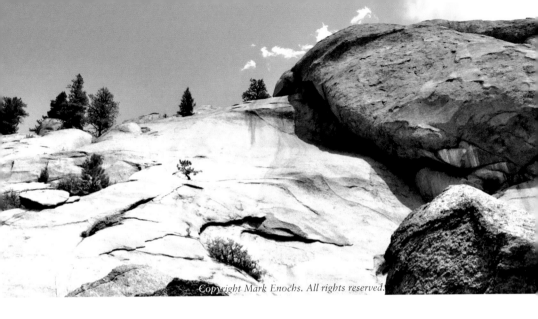

TAKE THE HIGH ROAD

—Marla Salmon

"When dealing with tough situations, there are three things you must remember: vision, partnering, and courage. Always take the high road, even though this is often the tough road, and you will find more solid ground."

Courage and Conviction Discourage Discrimination

—Mary Elizabeth Carnegie

During the 1940s, Elizabeth, as she was called, an African-American nurse, was informed that if she spoke at the national nursing convention, the White nurses would walk out. She did speak, and no one walked out.

We must all face our fears head-on to truly understand what defines a strong leader. The message Elizabeth imparted to her audience that day may have been so compelling they chose to stay and listen rather than walk out—assuming the White nurses ever seriously intended to walk out. But she never would have known had she not faced her fear head-on and pro-actively. Elizabeth learned to trust in the power of her message to overcome obstacles placed in her path, including intimidating tactics, and she experienced the positive impact of leadership by standing up to and facing down discrimination and intimidation.

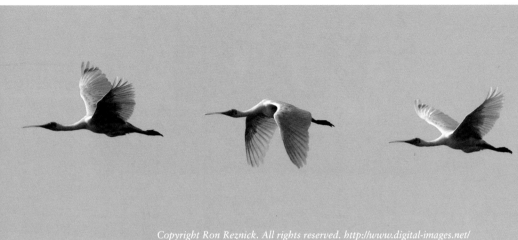

LEADERSHIP PACE

—Loretta Ford

"Be in a hurry; there is not a moment to waste. I make mistakes and correct them before they are even noticed. Besides, it is difficult to hit a moving target."

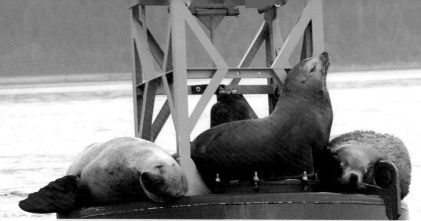

WEIGHING IN

—Marla Salmon

"There is a world of apathy out there. Every single day there are many things that aren't right. While you have to pick your battles, it is very important that when you encounter things that aren't right, you weigh in on them. Leadership is learning how to do that effectively. You won't be a reasonable leader if you don't have the instinct to say: *'This is something I have to put right.'*"

Can you identify anything in your work environment that isn't "right" and would be worthy of a battle? Are there individual, unit, organizational, or community barriers to teamwork or outcomes? Who would you need to enlist in changing the attitude and energy around the accepted apathy?

32

DISPARITY OF OPINION

—Luther Christman

"Nursing is being watered down with the different entry levels, thus making the profession weaker." Throughout his entire career, Luther was passionate about moving all nurses toward graduate-level education. Many of his bold and challenging sentiments were not embraced by other nurse leaders, but he strived for what he believed in and continues to do so today.

He shared his passionate voice and ideas with nursing colleagues, but he was not always popular. His direct manner of raising the bar on the profession offended some. Luther could look at other health care professions and see what nursing lacked. His outspokenness provoked strong reactions that made him feel persecuted for being a man—a minority—in nursing. The differences of opinion were polarizing enough to create an insurmountable obstacle to his aspirations to achieve the highest offices in nursing organizations.

Have you ever withheld your opinion because it was different from the mainstream opinion? What made you reluctant to speak your mind? Could you have found words that would have expressed your opinion in a collaborative manner?

LIVING THE LESSONS

—Kirsten Stallknecht

"I learned by *doing* my entire career."

As a young president of the powerful Danish Nursing Organization in a country with universal health care, there were times Kirsten was publicly chastised in the mainstream media for her missteps. This would be difficult for any leader, but it was especially challenging for a *young* novice. When she fumbled in making a decision, she learned from her mistake and strategized more effective methods the next time around. Kirsten never gave up, and she showed tremendous perseverance at any job or task she undertook. She learned that although change was often slow, if tackled with realistic expectations, it would be deliberate and effective.

There are textbooks to teach everything from A to Z, but nothing replaces the applied lessons learned from firsthand experience. While some students are "book smart," it is the learning, fumbling, and relearning that create opportunities for lasting lessons.

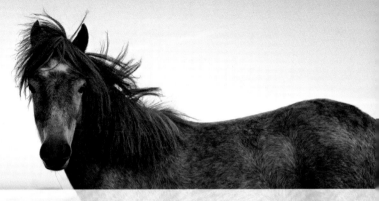

Don't Take It Personally

—*Dr. Sue Kushal*

Leaders often have to make decisions that aren't popular. "People will counter and question you. I would advise taking a deep breath and then responding to the issue. Never take it personally. This is so important as a leader. Sometimes people mean it personally and sometimes they don't, but, regardless, I don't play that game. I don't take it personally, so I don't respond in a personal manner to someone. I think you only hurt relationships in that case."

REJECT FIVE-YEAR PLANS

—Marla Salmon

"I don't believe in five-year plans. I think they make you work toward jobs instead of commitments." Commonly, a job is defined by words and a limited scope of expectation. It can be as simple as what one does to earn a paycheck. A commitment is driven by passion. The boundaries for fulfilling a commitment are fluid, dynamic, and limitless. Commitments are something you believe in and live for. What are your commitments?

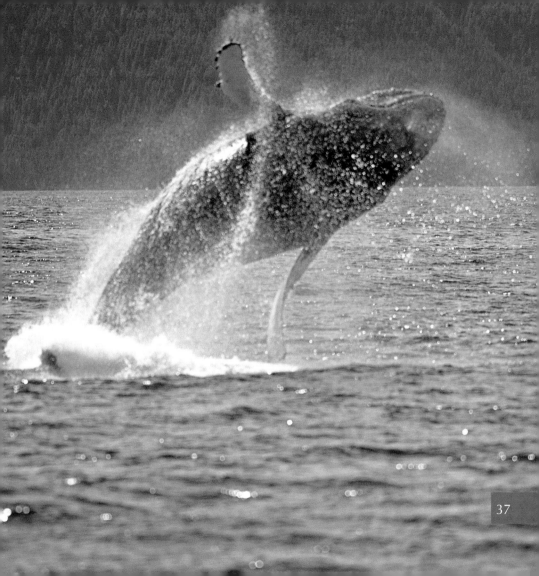

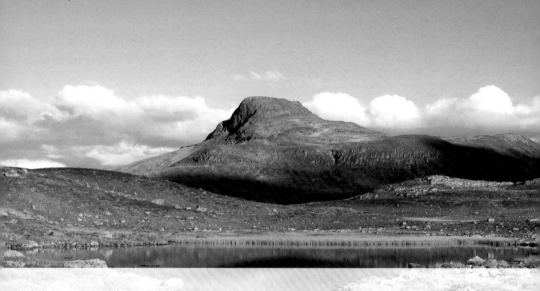

No Money, No Mission

Kristen Stallknecht

"You are never free if at the mercy of weak finances." All organizations have financial challenges, but some have more than others. Leaders can find their hands tied in decision making because resources are so scarce. The leader must ensure fiscal viability, or the overarching vision will ultimately fail.

LOSING IS PART OF LEADERSHIP, TOO

—Ada Sue Hinshaw

A leader must be "comfortable playing the game and not always winning." When pioneering new professional pathways, "you sometimes stumble, because there are no histories or rules to abide by."

When Ada Sue participated in the development of the National Center for Nursing Research at the National Institutes of Health, there was no history to guide her leadership. The American Nurses Association and prominent nurse researchers worked tirelessly to secure House and Senate passage to add the center. President Reagan vetoed it, not once, but twice. The House and Senate then voted overwhelmingly to override the second presidential veto. Ada Sue and her colleagues finally stumbled across the finish line, making history and rules as they went.

Reflect on a time when you were asked to create the history and rules as you went. How do you respond to losing when you have given your best effort to achieving a worthy victory?

GET WHAT YOU DESERVE

—Vernice Ferguson

Vernice found two phrases that were key motivators in guiding her career choices: "Never take a back seat," and "Never take 'no' for an answer." She never believed nurses should take the back seat to physicians nor accept anything less than what was offered to physicians—including her salary as chief nurse at the National Institutes of Health!

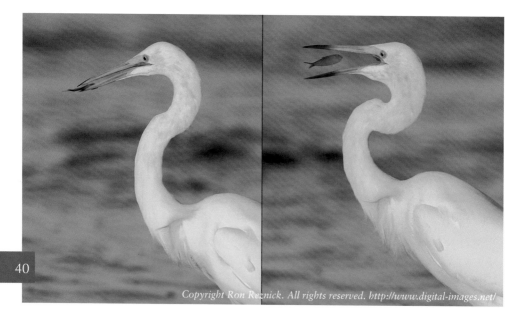

COME BACK STRONGER

—Faye Abdellah

"Overcoming the fear of taking a risk and failing is one of life's most valuable lessons. Where most will give up, a leader will come back stronger.""

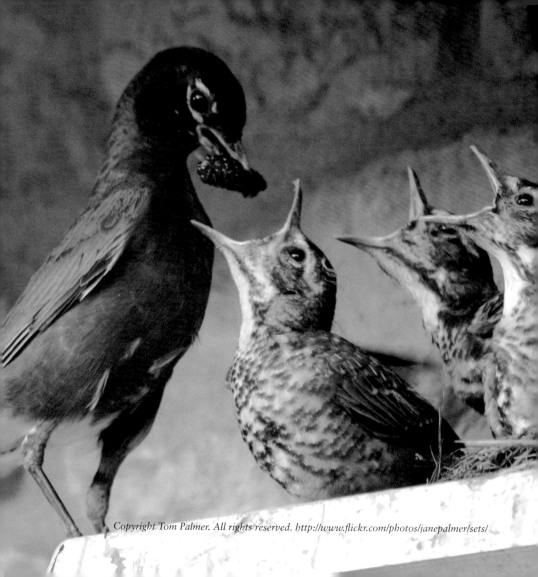

3

Developing the Next Generation of Leaders

Development of the next generation of leaders must be purposeful and part of our daily leadership responsibilities. Investing in the professional growth of up-and-coming leaders is the only way that nursing can continue to gain professional status and influence at all levels of health care delivery, from the bedside to international forums. All of us wish we had a wise person in our life to guide us on the most difficult of days—someone who could coach us to productive leadership and show us our blind spots in a safe manner, while demanding a higher level of performance.

How many times have you asked yourself, *"What would Florence Nightingale (or some other leadership hero) have done in this situation?"* This section offers some answers to that question, providing tips from the wisest of leaders whose legacies and lessons to the profession continue to live on. The following passages share insights and wisdom on attributes that can be used along your journey toward developing into a leader of influence. The lessons address a variety of professional development issues—responsibility to the profession, how to deal with rejection, becoming an agent of change, leaving a legacy, advice on when to step away from a position, and mentoring others in the profession—to name but a few.

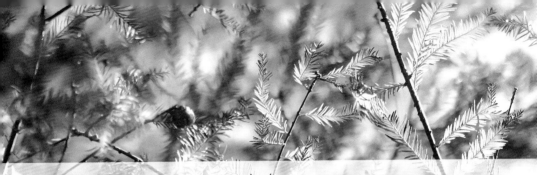

LEADERSHIP MOTIVATION

—Marla Salmon

"I never wanted to become anything. I wanted to *do* things that mattered—things that fundamentally haunt you—like the faces of migrant children, or the shoes on the beach in Sri Lanka [post Indonesian tsunami], things that have social meaning and importance."

Her passion to do things that mattered led Marla to assume leadership roles where she had the ability to find solutions. Marla may have never intended to be a member of the 48th World Health Organization or the chief nurse of the United States, but she didn't waste a moment in creating positive and necessary change when she got to these influential positions.

LEAVING A LEGACY

—Vernice Ferguson

Vernice believed in the power of mentoring. She created a mentoring program within the Veterans Administration Hospital system after observing that nurses were placed in leadership roles without the proper training and mentoring, yet they were expected to succeed. Vernice encouraged nurses to advance their careers, but she also created learning opportunities for nurses with high potential to learn upper-level management and leadership skills. Her goal was to help shape their growth as professionals. It was her way of giving back to nurses and the profession. "To have nurses actualized through my office, my resources, and through me, so they could continue to grow and be whatever they wanted to be in nursing, is just one way of giving back." Vernice believes that "educators, researchers, and administrators will find their way along, but the young need the extra guidance and extended hand of our profession's more senior and experienced colleagues."

The term "mentor" can be used in a formal manner when indicating a relationship that was established with clear goals and parameters for guidance and support for the mentee. At other times, a mentor can be more informal and include friends, colleagues, or others whom you lean on as a professional sounding board. Whom do you go to when needing professional support? Do you consider that person to be your mentor?

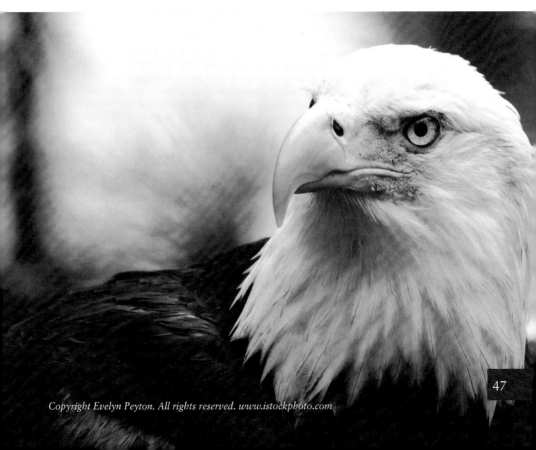

FIND YOUR PASSION

—Claire Fagin

"One must be visible in fighting for what one is passionate about, and hope the rest will follow." Most leaders can look over their shoulders and know others are following. Passion is part of the charisma that defines a strong leader.

What about the nursing profession makes you passionate? Can you remember why you decided to be a nurse? Does that fire still burn inside you?

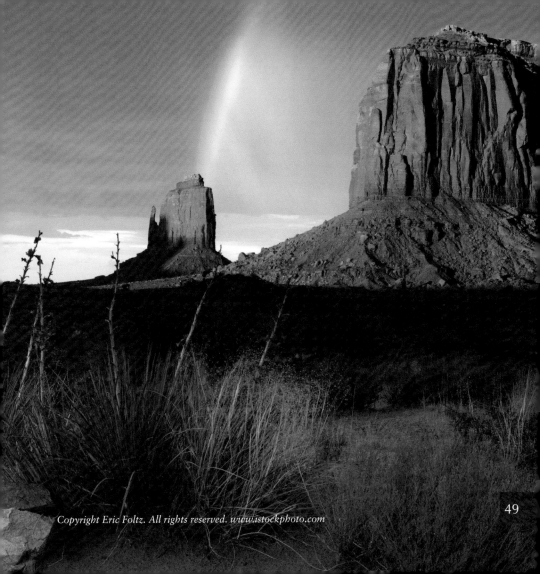

49

ON BEING PRESENT AND POWERFUL

—Loretta Ford

"Get to the table and be a player, or someone who doesn't understand nursing will do that for you."

This statement involves two distinct mandates: getting the right people to the table and being prepared to make a difference once there. It is then the responsibility of the leader—executive or bedside—to make their contributions indispensable to the process. This relates to the second point of being a player.

In a health care world of infinite needs and finite resources, being a player means knowing *how* to make the case using rigorous and meaningful data to demonstrate outcomes—patient, financial, employee, and community. Being a player means presenting the "so what" of the situation in a way that is compelling and salient. Coming to the table prepared and confident is essential to making contributions.

One example of this is nurse staffing ratios. If nursing is unwilling or unable to make the business case for adequate nurse staffing, then the chief financial officer (CFO) will most assuredly and independently make this budget decision, perhaps without the correct and necessary information. This may be a case of "not knowing what they don't know" rather than holding back resources. Decisions will be made with or without you, so how do you make sure that the right people are at the table and that they are effective players once there?

THE ABILITY TO CREATE CHANGE

—Claire Fagin

"Many times nurses don't feel they are in a position to make change, but I want them to understand that nurses can make change happen, providing they have both persistence and visibility for their work." Look around at how nurses effect change every day and realize how you can, too. Claire Fagin did this through the power of her dissertation, which studied the effects of parents on the recovery outcomes of hospitalized children. From these observations, the concept of "rooming in" was born. Claire's research changed pediatric nursing and pediatric patient care.

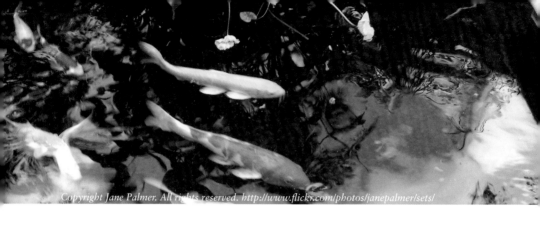

SELECTING THE TEAM

—Ada Sue Hinshaw

Leaders know it is important to "get good people around you, people who complement your strengths and people who will tell you 'no.'"

The team should exemplify that the sum is greater than the individual parts. When hiring new team members, it is important to know what talent you have and what talent you must seek to meet the organization's strategic plan. A team that replicates talent and doesn't respectfully engage in debate is a team with limitations. Experienced leaders will hire direct reports who are brighter and more talented than they are. Have you ever heard the saying that the 9s will hire 10s and the 7s will hire 6s? Watch for the pattern. In which category do you fit?

Respecting and Facilitating the Vision

—Joyce Clifford

Joyce knows what she did best: "I built great leaders, and those leaders created excellence." Those who worked with Joyce described her as someone who set the standards and expectations and then allowed others to create the outcomes. Her gift has always been the vision. She set the vision and then got out of the way and let those with the most knowledge create the reality. She always made sure that she presented a dream that was feasible, with resources that were available.

Joyce was so successful at building great leaders that to date, 11 of her protégés have become chief nursing officers at hospitals across the United States.

BEDSIDE NURSES KNOW

—Linda Aiken

In calling bedside nurses to leadership roles and responsibilities, Linda states that "many of the most important research issues in nursing come from clinicians who are the closest to the patients, and they need to figure out a way to articulate these issues. They do not necessarily have to do the research, but must be willing to speak and write about what these important problems are" to drive the research.

—Faye Abdellah

Faye Abdellah realized nurses had Nobel Prize-winning ideas but not the research knowledge to develop the initial premise. Faye recalls that a bedside nurse first observed that 100% oxygen given to premature infants might be associated with blindness. The nurse did not know how to take the observation forward into a research study. However, a non-nursing researcher did research the topic and won the Nobel Prize. The Nobel Prize might have gone to a nurse, if she had moved the bedside knowledge to research practice.

Go With the Flow—You Never Know Where It Will Take You

—Linda Aiken

"I didn't know I wanted to be a researcher, but a big part of my education at the University of Florida emphasized that nursing should be evidence-based." Long before evidence-based practice became the standard, Linda was interested in clinical problems, such as postoperative psychosis after heart surgery. Because she knew little about the research process, she partnered with a clinical psychologist to learn how to conduct a clinical trial. Linda's research career was launched, and she became a major contributor to evidence-based practice in health care today.

ON REJECTION

—Judith Shamian

"Rejection is a part of leadership." As a relatively new nurse (30 years old) attempting to step into key leadership roles, Judith was turned down the first several times she applied. Through perseverance, though, she received a promotion that helped shape her career. The rise did not come overnight, but Judith's talents were recognized and rewarded over time. She stepped into a director-level position and was the youngest among her senior-ranking contemporaries in the hospital. Judith knew she was talented and never allowed herself to become discouraged. Her faith in her own abilities paid off.

Rejection is something we all face, even early in life. Were you chosen last for a sports team in school? Some use those painful moments of rejection to find the fortitude needed to persevere and try again. Have you ever been rejected or passed over in an area you later came back to with great success? Don't give up because you were rejected: Reflect and rethink your goals.

SPANNING THE PROFESSION

—Gretta Styles

"I consider myself a *professionalist*, which is a term that I coined. It is some-one who wants to develop the profession, all aspects of it. One is not just a researcher, educator, or practitioner, but interested in developing all aspects of those to meet the criteria of a profession."

AN UNEXPECTED GIFT TO NURSING

—Marla Salmon

"The nursing shortage has been a real gift to nursing. A lot of people are talking about nursing who didn't talk about nursing before." The next generation of nurses will have opportunities to be a part of the workforce shortage solution. Enjoy the bright light of attention and take advantage of the leadership that will be provided to you to find solutions.

KNOWING WHEN TO STEP ASIDE

—Loretta Ford and Joyce Clifford

In 2005, Loretta and Joyce sat in an audience while a spirited debate raged about the purpose and importance of two emerging roles in nursing: the doctor of nursing practice (DNP) and clinical nurse leader (CNL). In the 1960s, Loretta had led the development of the then-new role of nurse practitioner. In the 1970s, Joyce had crafted the professional practice model with responsibilities similar to the CNL. Both Loretta and Joyce sat in silence throughout the debate. When asked on separate occasions about their silence, both responded nearly identically, stating: "This is a conversation that must occur amongst the contemporary leadership; it is their debate, not mine. If asked, I will help sort out *their* ideas." Knowing when to step away is also a key leadership lesson.

By stepping aside at the right moment, leaders can build the confidence of the new generation of leaders. This passing of the leadership torch allows for contemporary leaders to step out from the shadow of the giants and create energy that builds on history, but allows for a new direction. Can you reflect on a time when you inspired an idea, but the front-line work of others modified and operationalized the idea into a superior outcome?

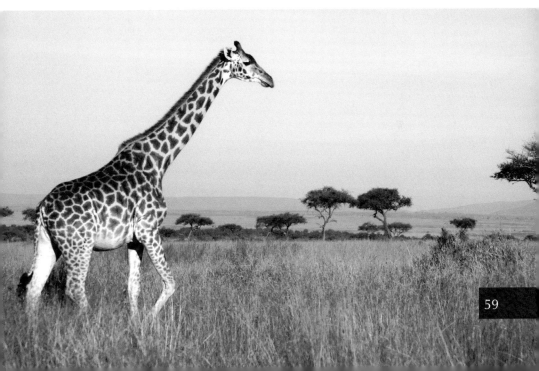

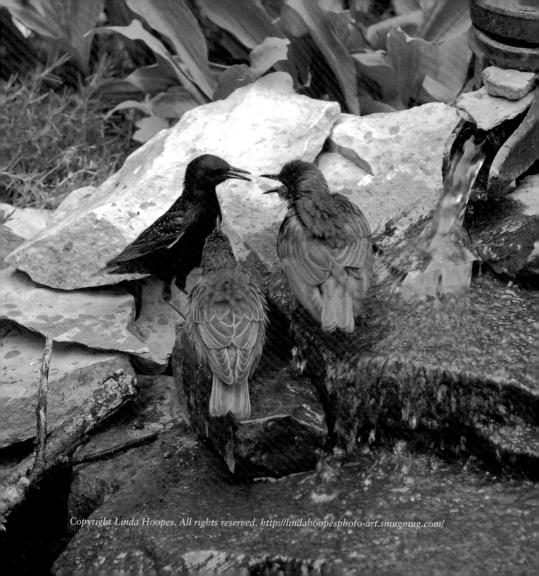

Communicating the Message

Strong communication skills are key tools for leaders, regardless of profession or industry. The ability to provide clarity of vision and motivate others to their maximum potential defines the leader. It is relatively easy to lead when times are good and momentum within an organization is steady. When times are most unstable, though, it is the leader who must provide the confidence and clarity of vision. Good communicators make one want to line up behind them and follow wherever they might be going. Their message is passionate and heartfelt, articulate and clear. Their authenticity and willingness to lead make us want to serve under them, because they are skilled at communicating the message.

Leaders are in positions to communicate messages that either do or don't impact the lives of those around them. Think about your work experiences, and remember the leaders who helped transition organizations through rough times of change. Strong leaders choose their words deliberately and prepare carefully when communicating key messages. The following words of wisdom show how these pivotal leaders have leveraged their voice to influence change and impact those around them.

ON CONFLICT

—Joyce Clifford

"Conflict is OK and sometimes necessary. Unresolved conflict is NOT!"

TAKING RESPONSIBILITY AND CONDUCTING THE "ORCHESTRA"

—Rheba de Tornyay

As the dean at the University of Washington, Rheba understood there would be times of controversy, and she knew it was her job to bring the team together. She understood that "trying to please everyone meant pleasing no one." The buck had to stop somewhere, and it was with her. Rheba managed this responsibility through exquisite communication. Her colleagues describe Rheba as one of the great conductors of communication in the profession. She worked diligently to get the players on the same page—playing at the same tempo and generating enthusiasm for the performance. She had the power to persuade leaders outside of nursing to hear and appreciate the music. Good leaders must learn to be great conductors.

COMMUNICATE
EFFECTIVELY SO OTHERS
FOLLOW

—Vernice Ferguson

Vernice learned firsthand the power of communication among staff nurses. Once, Vernice had been sure she spoke for all nurses on her staff when she suggested a change in procedure that was intended to help the nurses. Strangely, the nurses did not support her when a physician went behind her back to survey her staff on how *they* felt about her proposed changes. When she confronted the nurses, she realized that while she spoke *for* them, she had not spoken *with* them and given them a chance to be heard.

"I learned how to lead better from my earlier mistake of thinking I had the followers with me and discovered that when the heat was on, they could not be counted on to be supportive." On a second occasion, Vernice specifically went around the table person by person to have each of them weigh in on the issue under discussion. This time, each could leave the room and know he or she was part of the final decision.

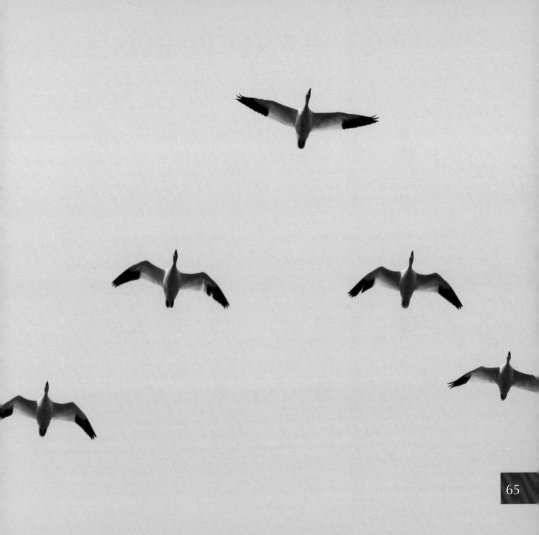

LET IT GO—AND PUBLISH

—Linda Aiken

Linda is recognized as one of nursing's most prolific writers. It wasn't always easy. "For me, writing is a love/hate thing, and though I have gotten better at it, it is still very hard to write. No pain, no gain: If you want to see change in nursing, then you must get ideas to the profession through publication." When Linda was asked about learning to write, she responded: "I learned to let go. I told myself that these are ideas that need to get into print, so that someone else can make them better. Don't expect to later look back on publications and see perfection. I have become a better writer over time."

The first steps in writing are:

- Know what you want to say,
- Conduct the research, and
- Put words on the page.

Once you have your ideas on paper, step away, clear your mind, and read it with a fresh perspective. Ask yourself:

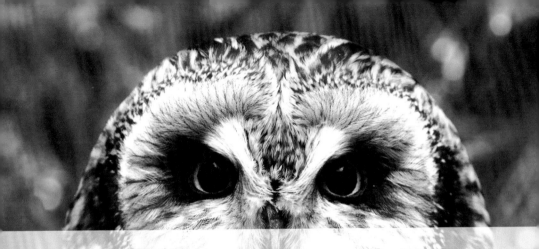

- Does it say what I want it to say?
- Does it make sense and have a logical flow?
- Is the topic clear and compelling?
- Would I be interested in reading this?
- Does it make a contribution?

If you can answer yes to these questions, it is time to send it out for an objective critique. Give it to someone who is knowledgeable and will unabashedly tell you the truth with the genuine intent of improving the paper. Then, as Linda indicated, "let go" of it and give the ideas to the profession for a broader review and reactions. What comes back will be better because of the power of collective thought.

GETTING AND REMEMBERING THE MESSAGE

—Margaret McClure

"I don't think it is possible for anybody to become over-prepared in communication skills; this contributes greatly to professional success. You have to be able to organize what you need to deliver, and to deliver it in a way that people are going to get it and remember it."

Leaders should devise methods to evaluate if the intended message was received and remembered. This may require multiple inputs and methods to ascertain if more communication on the subject is needed or the point was made the first time. Close the loop on communication.

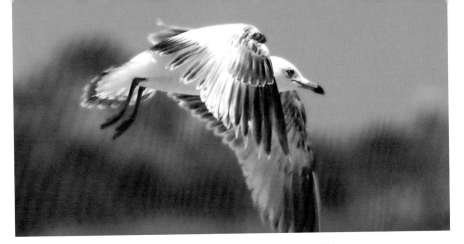

DIRECTION WITH DIGNITY

—Luther Christman

"Many of the communication problems that exist among physicians and nurses relate to the level of education among nurses. Knowledge is power, and professional learning is a lifelong commitment to learning."

As harsh as these words may sound, Luther is one of the profession's strongest advocates for maintaining the dignity of nurses. There is an art to delivering the strong message while maintaining the dignity of others—they must hear the direction and respect the intent. This is the challenge to the leader—*direction with dignity*.

How to Write a Complete Sentence

—Margaret McClure

"One of nursing's biggest handicaps is that we are in a field where your basic practice requires that you never write in a complete sentence. Nurses need to learn how to write. Writing is the kind of thing you get better at as you do it; you have to practice to improve. However, don't be fooled—just because someone has a PhD doesn't mean they can write."

When writing a collaborative piece, identify the writing strengths of the team and make assignments accordingly. Learn how to elicit the strengths of each team member and then edit to one voice. Writing can be intimidating, so make it fun by allowing everyone to shine. Ask everyone to check his or her ego at the door!

PREPARE THE MESSAGE

—Ada Sue Hinshaw

Always be prepared. When communicating the message, nurses need to be "more precise, more crisp, and more clinically relevant than anybody else; it is not different from any minority group making its niche."

SPEAK EARLY

—Linda Aiken

Linda was given this advice by a mentor: "Speak early in a meeting, because the ability to add creativity and innovation diminishes as the conversation progresses."

DRIVING THE MESSAGE

—Ada Sue Hinshaw

"Know your message and no matter what is asked, be sure you get your intended message across." The best way to accomplish this is to come prepared, which means role-playing your message with colleagues who will test your ability to stay on point and say it clearly.

When Ada Sue was delivering her nursing research message to Congress, she told them what she wanted them to know. They didn't know what nursing research was or why they should care. It was her job to drive the message and not allow the message to get off-track. This is a skill that must be practiced to the point where it is subtle and effective.

BEING PRESENT IS
POWERFUL LEADERSHIP

—Shirley Chater

On 19 April 1995, Shirley Chater was thrust into a crisis after the Murrah Federal Building in Oklahoma City was bombed. She did not have answers for this situation; her nursing experience directed her actions.

"This incident was the most moving experience of my career. My role was to establish the fact very forcefully that leadership from the top was present and doing something about the situation, and most importantly, to make sure families were being cared for."

The need to make leadership visible applies in every setting. In this example, the key tool is how Shirley communicated she was present and available to families and employees. She didn't make big leadership actions or decisions, but just listened and cared enough to hear the hurt everyone was feeling.

REALIGN ACCOUNTABILITY FOR PREVENTIVE HEALTH CARE

—Richard Carmona

"The average person takes little responsibility for their own health. The majority of the disease burden in our society is preventable. The economic burden is therefore preventable. However, we live in a society that blindly says 'give me that.' The patient's liver fails after years of drug and alcohol abuse and they say, 'I want a new liver.' The patient's lungs fail after years of smoking and they say, 'I want a new lung.' We continue to pay for people who insist on drinking too much, smoking too much, driving too fast, engaging in high-risk activities, gaining weight, choosing a sedentary lifestyle, and the list goes on and on."

Future conversations about health care reform must incorporate and communicate a message of prevention and individual accountability.

CONNECT WITH THE AUDIENCE

—Margaret McClure

"The language you choose has to connect with the audience. For example, there are many churches to attend in New York City, but I go where the minister really has something to say from the pulpit. The rest of the service is fine, but I want to hear the scholarly part of the service; however, he can't preach as if he is a scholar. The minister has to use ordinary language that people appreciate, understand, and relate to—so must nurse leaders."

The staff must *feel* that you understand what the front line looks like, and active listening is the key to this end.

Nurses Should Be the Glue

—Marla Salmon

Marla has encountered nurses who make the mistake of "coming to the decision-making table as agenda bearers, as people who aren't willing to help others but want their help."

If invited to the decision-making table, nurses must be prepared to participate as a team member to address the global issues, not just nursing. To believe that only nursing should have a voice, or the loudest and most important voice, is myopic. Nursing has an important responsibility to be the glue maintaining the interdisciplinary conversation that will place the patient at the center of the discussion.

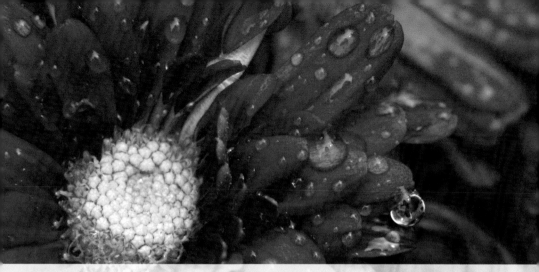

KEEP THE COMMUNICATION FOCUS ON PATIENTS

—Joyce Clifford

"Sometimes the leadership team can get bogged down in arguments over the opinions of the group, often driven by their discipline focus. The best thing to do at this point is ask for a 'time out' and refocus the conversation away from 'who is right' to 'what is the right thing to do for the patient and family.'"

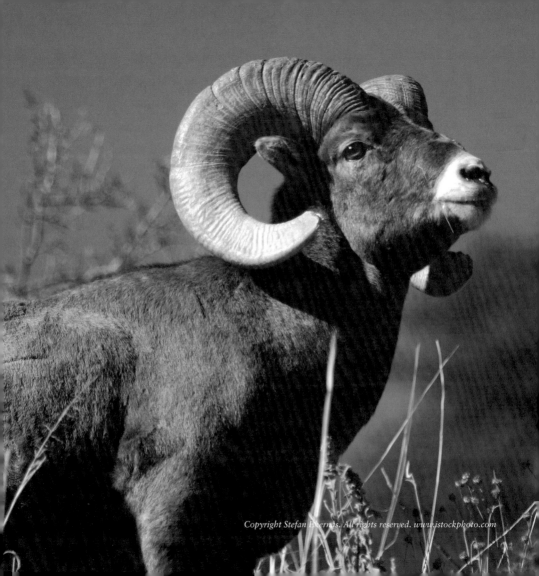

5

Integrity

The importance of integrity is underscored by Warren Buffet, chief executive officer of Berkshire Hathaway: "In looking for people to hire, you look for three qualities: integrity, intelligence, and energy. And if they don't have the first, the other two will kill you." (Buffet, 2006)

Integrity should be the guiding principle of one's leadership—the moral character and dependably honest nature of one's action. Choosing integrity creates the foundation for mutual respect and trust in relationships. Martin Luther King, Jr., stated that "the time is always right to do what is right." Maintaining one's integrity is easy when all is moving harmoniously.

However, when leadership faces high-stake challenges, conflict can erase years of integrity development. The algorithm for maintaining one's integrity can be found in the following poem by an anonymous author:

Be careful of your thoughts,
for your thoughts become your words;
Be careful of your words,
for your words become your deeds;
Be careful of your deeds,
for your deeds become your habits;
Be careful of your habits,
for your habits become your character;
Be careful of your character,
for your character becomes your destiny.

ACCESS TO CARE

—Ruth Lubic

"To pretend that health is somehow separate from people's social conditions is madness. No patient should be denied access to care, regardless of health status or insurance. That is the passionate message I believe and fight for every day of my professional career."

ETHICAL DILEMMAS
CHALLENGE INTEGRITY

—Leah Curtin

Ethical dilemmas commonly occur around questions of futile care. Leah reminds us that "care is never futile, but the medical intervention may be." She defines futile medical intervention as "anything that does not have a better than 1% chance of helping someone, and it has to be sustained by data."

How should futile care be managed? Should futile care be managed at all? Do you believe that medical interventions may be futile? If so, at what point does care become futile? Who should make these decisions—family, nurses, physicians, clergy, and/or courts?

THE SIMPLE VALUE OF RESPECT

—Shirley Chater

Shirley Chater was the first female assistant vice chancellor at the University of California, San Francisco, the first nurse president at Texas Woman's University, and the first nurse who became commissioner of the Social Security Administration (SSA) for the United States—with responsibility for 62,000 employees. She never lost sight of the simple values of cooperative leadership and respect for others.

No matter how big a role one plays within an organization, the values from which one operates can be very simple. Shirley entered a governmental agency that was accustomed to a *command and control environment*. The commissioner was expected to tell the employees what to do, and the employees would obey. This did not fit Shirley's leadership style. She managed to change the culture—over time, out of respect for her colleagues—into a

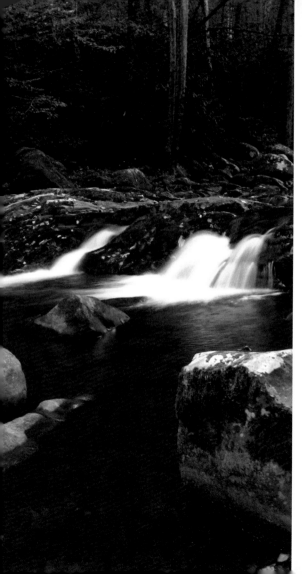

more cooperative and collaborative management style, where input from employees and customers was valued and taken into consideration. Shirley's leadership and basic values produced results that placed the SSA at the top of the list (Dalbar and Associates, 1995) in customer service excellence—ahead of Disney World!

DRAWING THE LINE IN THE SAND

—Leah Curtin

Leah defines integrity as "doing what you think is the right thing or, if you don't, at least admit it." She warns that when you are considering action provoked by a threat to integrity, do so with full knowledge that you will most likely do so alone. She states: "When you draw a line in the sand, understand it is your line, and it is your sand, and nobody else is going to defend that turf with you; you are on your own." Leah believes the biggest ethical challenge in most people's lives is trying to maintain integrity.

Leah was compelled by her professional integrity to question a physician who was prescribing excessive doses of medication for patients. She challenged organizational leaders to stop the practice. When confronted, she stood by her line in the sand to bring forward a physician practice that wasn't right, and she believed this should be acknowledged and stopped.

Her integrity meant more to her than her job, and she felt comfortable defending her turf. Can you think of a time when you should have defended your turf but didn't? Was there a time when you chose integrity and led significant change? Is that time now?

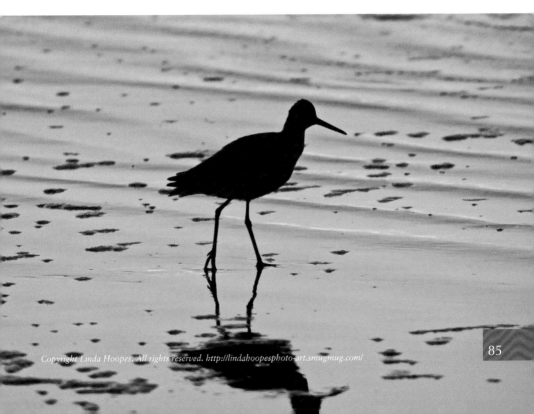

85

BRIDGES

—Marla Salmon

"The bridge you burn is the one you will have to cross later."

Marla is emphatic that leaders must approach conflict with "civility, which means engaging in and appreciating the differences—reciprocity starts with you."

A Japanese proverb states: "The reputation of a thousand years may be determined by the conduct of one hour." Inevitably, you will face leadership moments in which your words or actions do not reflect your true beliefs and standards. These regrettable leadership moments can occur at the most un-expected and inconvenient of times. A moment of restraint and an attitude of professionalism can determine if your future opportunities are maximized or minimized. Civility always pays off.

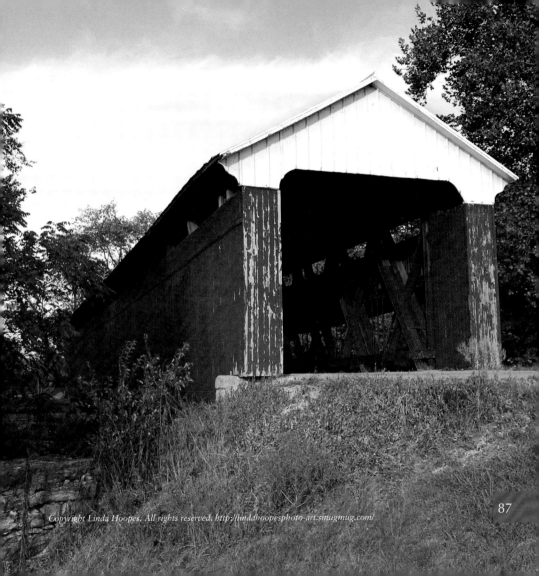

87

Do the Right Thing

—Richard Carmona

"Leadership in its simplest form is: You are responsible for the destiny of others. This is a very magnanimous responsibility and a humbling one, because you can't take it lightly. Good leaders understand that they must lead with integrity and dignity," which Rich defines as "doing the right thing when no one is watching, and recognizing the importance of the greater good while subordinating your own interests."

Accepting the Many Faces of "Right"

—Joyce Clifford

Tolerance for differences is essential in leadership. It is possible—in fact, probable—that more than one team member is "right." Joyce encourages leaders to listen to all ideas and create an environment of mutual respect for differences. Quite simply: Treat others as you wish to be treated. Live by the Golden Rule.

88

ABUSE OF POWER

—Judith Shamian

"A leader may have acquired power by the position they hold; however, not everyone uses power wisely."

Have you ever worked for someone who did not use power wisely? They made decisions in their own best interest, but not in the best interests of the organization. You found yourself asking why no one stepped in to say or do something about the injustice. The outcome of these situations is not good, and it comes down to assessing your own values and asking if you still are a good fit within the organization.

Managing Personal Ambitions

— Ruth Lubic

"Leaders have to learn to deal with people who are willing to sacrifice others to suit their personal ambitions. Even the best lessons can be difficult to learn sometimes."

In leadership, not everyone plays by the same rule book. Some leaders play fair, with a focus on the greater good. Other leaders will sacrifice their colleagues for personal gain and never look back. Understand the game you are in, and learn how you can maintain a focus on the professional outcome without becoming a victim.

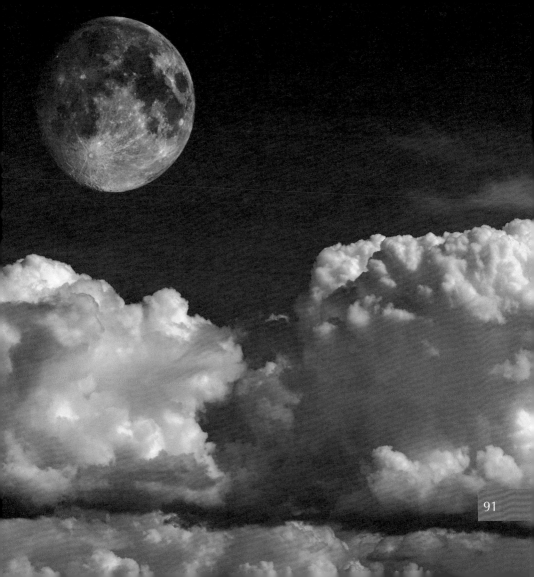

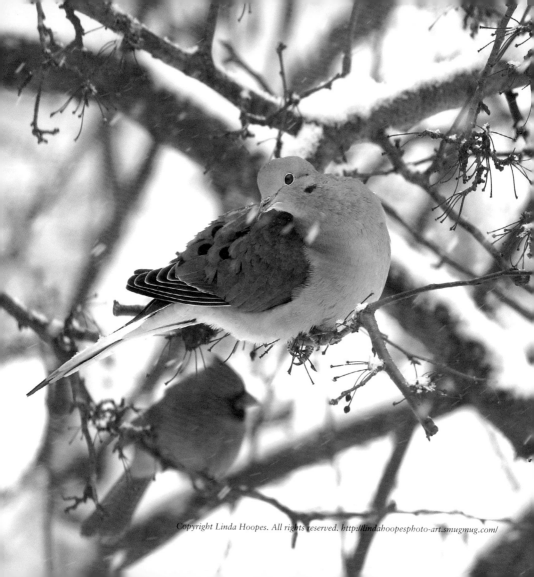

6

Political Acuity

Political acuity is the ability to navigate political realities to generate necessary support for fulfilling organizational goals, initiatives, and agendas. Understanding how the organizational culture operates can make the difference between a great idea soaring or crash-landing into flames. Sometimes the rules of engagement are transparent and relatively easy to navigate. At other times, unknown trolls lurk under the bridge with an agenda that promises to erode your leadership influence. Even building one's leadership credibility within an organization means understanding the accepted method of leading. Is it building relationships before dealing with issues? Or, is it dealing with issues as a means of developing relationships? Each organization has an institutional memory that was built around many years of culture. The leader must adapt a style to facilitate leadership influence.

Leaders can be frustrated and demoralized by political acuity dead-ends. These leadership lessons help provide insight, perspective, and encouragement around issues of political acuity.

Don't Give Away Leadership Opportunities

—Florence Wald

"I hired a consultant for the first hospice in the United States to obtain a certificate of need and to navigate the rules and regulations, which I didn't understand. Within 18 months, he had convinced the board to seek my resignation. I refused, and they had to fire me. At one point, I was asked to consider a board position, but I was concerned that I wasn't qualified because I was a nurse. At that time, nurses serving on a board was not commonplace. I had the ability, but I didn't have the sense of responsibility, and I didn't survive." Florence regrets "giving away this leadership opportunity."

Always be aware of what you may be giving away. Think carefully about this before you reject opportunities out of hand.

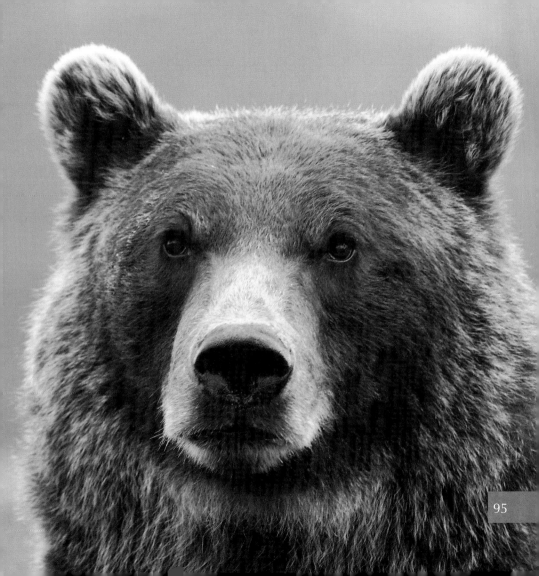

POLITICS EQUALS PARTNERSHIP

—Ada Sue Hinshaw

Political acuity is dependent on strategic and ongoing communication. Ada Sue recalls the American Nurses Association (ANA) partnering with Congressman Edward Madigan to amend the National Institutes of Health (NIH) preauthorization legislation to allow for the creation of a new Institute of Nursing. Energy and excitement among nursing leaders were high as this important nursing research bill moved forward. Unfortunately, the ANA forgot to discuss the addition of a new institute with the NIH. Ada Sue candidly admits this was a major strategic blunder, as partnering with the NIH should have occurred early in the process. The bill failed on the first attempt. The lesson was learned the hard way and rectified before the second attempt.

Mingling Matters

—Ada Sue Hinshaw

You have to position yourself strategically and build strong relationships to create opportunities. From the beginning, Ada Sue knew that the National Center for Nursing Research (NCNR) at the National Institutes of Health (NIH) would one day be campaigning for full institute status. Her job, as the first director of the NCNR, was not only to build the science infrastructure of nursing, but also to personally develop the relationships that could promote program legitimacy. Ada Sue's best leadership decision was to live on the NIH campus and become part of the NIH family. Influential decision-makers came to know her integrity through channels outside the office. The discussions to move the NCNR from center to institute status eventually occurred at a cocktail party with Ada Sue's neighbors and friends, who knew her as a person and professional and trusted her judgment.

CHOOSE YOUR BOSS
CAREFULLY

—Marla Salmon

"Choose your boss carefully. You have to be on the same page with your boss, or the most attractive situation can become miserable. Look for a sense of connectedness and also a mutual agreement on the vision for the organization." This has a direct correlation on your quality of life. There are too many external battles to take on internal executive battles. Choose wisely.

ON CONVERGENCE
LEADERSHIP

—Marla Salmon

"I don't believe in consensus leadership—you wear people down in achieving consensus. I believe you lose what people have to offer that may be different by doing that. I believe in convergence leadership, where you identify points of common ground that naturally converge, such as quality of care, patient safety, patient satisfaction, and then you work from that vantage point by engaging in partnered ways."

THE INNER CIRCLE

Vernice Ferguson

It was always Vernice's quest to be at the table. The one question she always asked—whether in her role as nurse leader of the Veterans Administration Medical Center or chief nurse at the National Institutes of Health—was, "Where does the power lie?" Her response was always, "Be there. So, by hook or by crook, I was always in the inner circle. You position yourself to be in the inner circle, so that you can facilitate nursing in its fullness to have its day in the sun."

Have you ever been in meetings where key people speak up, and everyone hangs on every word they say? These individuals seem to command the respect of the group, whether or not they have the title to match. This is one tip in finding where the power lies: Just listen and watch.

KNOW YOUR CHIEF EXECUTIVE

—Margaret McClure

"Choose your nurse executive job based on the chief executive officer (CEO). You could say this is obvious, but it isn't that obvious to many people. If the CNO is fired, the next question should be, where is the CEO? The answer, more often than not, is that he or she just assumed leadership in the last year." The CEO is heavily dependent on the CNO, and the new CEO will often recruit or bring with him or her the CNO of his or her choosing. Understand that it isn't personal, and be strategic in your planning.

101

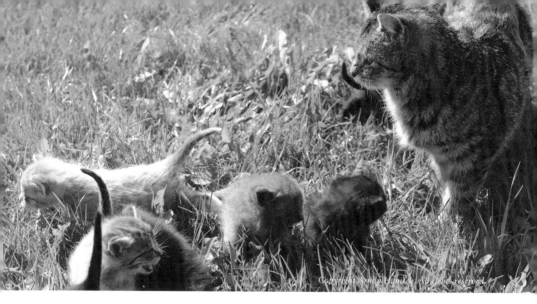

CAT HERDING

—Loretta Ford

When dealing with large-scale projects, it is essential to influence the masses to move together toward and with the change. Many leaders describe this as "cat herding." Loretta's recipe for success is: "Get some catnip, get in the middle of the circle, and make them come to you." Find out what is important to them and draw them in to the process, rather than aimlessly chasing those who enjoy the sport of chaos.

THE HOSPITAL'S CORE BUSINESS IS NURSING

—Margaret McClure

"Patients have always been admitted to the hospital because they need nurses. If they don't need professional monitoring by nurses, then almost everything can be done outpatient. We need to help hospital administrators understand that their core business is nursing. They are not in the medical business. Physicians are private entrepreneurs, their patients the customers. Often, even the physicians understand that hospitals are about nursing care and choose to stay because the nursing division meets their customer needs."

PARTNER WITH NURSES

—Richard Carmona

"The one thing I always told all the new residents is that the best thing you can do is befriend the nurses. They will educate you, and they will protect you. Remember, you are there for 5-10 minutes and nurses are there 24 hours a day. They are the true caregivers, and we come along and give episodic care."

103

Follow the Strings

—Marla Salmon

"Leaders must learn to challenge themselves and engage in constant discovery. Follow the strings and basically don't settle for the immediate explanation. Everything has obvious drivers, and beyond that are drivers that aren't so obvious but often are the root cause of what is really happening."

During one hospital's Magnet journey, leadership barriers emerged. Initially, hospital leaders clearly committed fiscal and human resources to become designated as a Magnet hospital. Yet, shortly into the journey, executive pushback and discomfort became obvious. The stated explanation was discord around suggested organizational change.

Following the strings allowed for the discovery that nearly a decade earlier the hospital leaders, who remained in power, had built its culture on an egalitarian foundation. The Magnet Recognition Program highlighted and diverted large financial resources to the nursing division—a significant and uncomfortable culture shift for this hospital. Understanding the driver

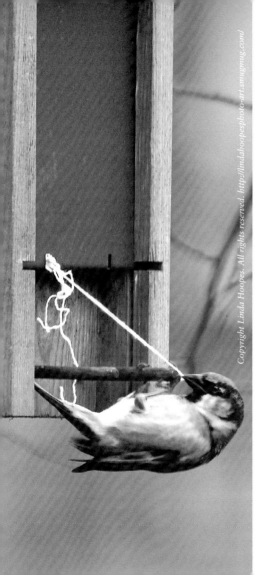

of resistance allowed for the creation of a Magnet culture that was interdisciplinary. The focus shifted away from Magnet and toward patient care excellence, which is something everyone could support. When the Magnet designation was announced, the celebration was attended by as many interdisciplinary colleagues as nurses. Following the strings allowed for success.

Nursing Budgets

—Margaret McClure

"Be comfortable with the fact that the nursing budget is always under attack. The nursing budget is the best controlled budget in the hospital, because it is so darn big. It is the best controlled budget because it is *always* under attack, and the administrator who is responsible for the nursing budget understands it better than the other administrators understand their budgets, just that simple."

The Power of Negotiating

—Judith Shamian

"I knew that whoever held the money held the power, and it was the key to negotiating."

ENOUGH SAID

—Mary Elizabeth Carnegie

"Times and people do change."

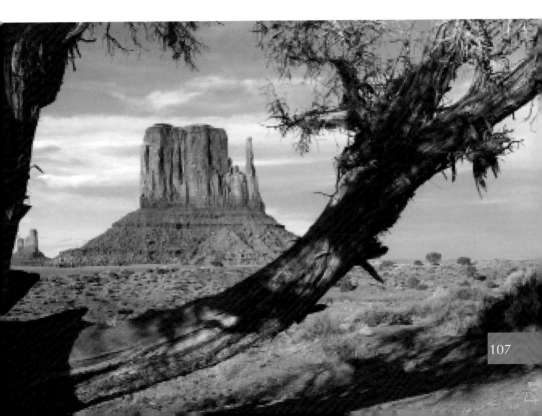

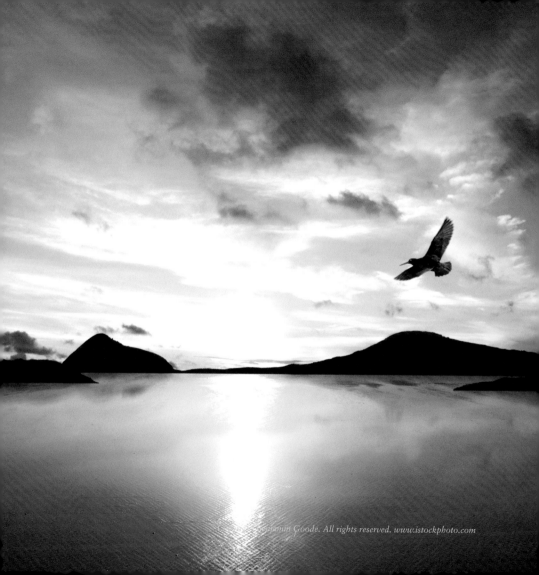

7

Golden Leadership Moments

There are moments in each leadership journey where it all seems to come together. The energy, desire, and attitude for a vision perfectly align with the trends of the time to produce an outcome that sometimes surprises everyone by the magnitude of its impact. Often these golden moments have been evolving across years of discovery and angst, times when the leader never gave up. These turning points in personal and professional history may be remembered as the inertia that preceded a paradigm shift—a different way of thinking or acting that improved the greater good. Risk taking and visionary thinking are fundamental elements for achieving golden leadership moments.

Golden leadership moments can also occur on a more individual level. You don't have to change the face of health care to experience golden leadership moments. These can be experiences when you have a breakthrough moment—the "ah-ha!" moment—resulting in a change in relationships, processes, or vision that opens up new pathways. These golden leadership moments are easily recalled with great pride as defining career moments.

NOT JUST A NURSE

—Margaret McClure

"I hear nurses say, 'I am just a nurse.' Can you imagine that? The most important person in a hospital and we discount our value. Nurses are the cornerstone of health care, and yet *they* don't respect what they do."

Nurses should be saying, "Look at me—I AM A NURSE," and demand that others in health care treat them with the respect they are due.

ON TIMING

"Patience in timing may not be wasted time."

Florence spent much of her early career feeling as if she didn't "fit" with the culture of patient care that commonly excluded patients from the process. For example, patients were not permitted to know their cancer diagnosis. They were fundamentally robbed of the ability to participate in decision-making or prepare for death. Florence was frustrated by the lack of patient-centered care in nursing and considered leaving the profession.

Years later, Florence heard Cicely Saunders speak about hospice care in England, and she knew that this was the nursing care model she had been seeking. The years of waiting for a culture to fit her beliefs may not have been wasted time. She grew as a leader, and she now had the networking and skills to establish hospice care in America.

Reflect on a time when a great idea didn't take off the first time it was presented but, with the passage of time, it was embraced and adopted when circumstances changed. What made the difference? How long did you have to wait? How did you develop your idea during the hiatus?

THE POWER OF ONGOING DEBATE

—Sue Donaldson

In 1970, Sue Donaldson and Dorothy Crowley began a daily cafeteria debate around the question of "what is the discipline of nursing?" "I had concluded that nursing did not have a discipline—I couldn't state it, nor could anyone else I knew," Sue says. Nursing doctoral programs across the nation were being rejected because of this problem. By chance and serendipity, Sue and Dorothy found themselves presenting the framework that defined the discipline of nursing as the keynote speakers at the 1977 Western Interstate Council for Higher Education in Nursing (WICHEN). When the session was finished, the room fell silent. Attendees were stunned by what they heard. This golden moment enabled nurse leaders to finally articulate to academia and other disciplines the distinct nature of the discipline of nursing.

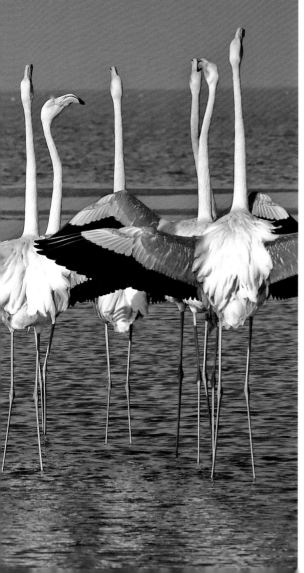

The Donaldson and Crowley paper has been successfully cited as justification for PhD programs in nursing. The number of PhD programs increased from fewer than eight in the mid-1970s to 83 in 2004. "We were not doing anything special," Sue says. "It was years of free thinking and debate without deadlines and boundaries, which had no real meaning at the time." Don't underestimate the power of scholarly debate, even when casual and open-ended.

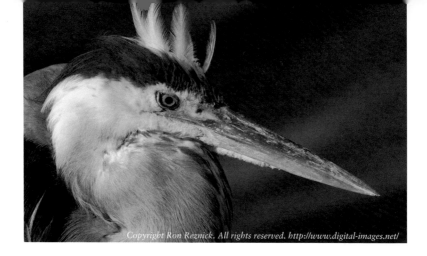

THE BURDEN OF SUCCESS

—Rheba de Tornyay

When Rheba announced to a classroom full of first-year students that "the University of Washington School of Nursing has been voted number one again," she recalls that they looked like "deer in headlights." Rheba laughed and remarked, "Your confidence in your school underwhelms me; what is the matter with you?" What she heard next surprised and shocked her. They were intimidated by the ranking and understood the burden imposed on them to maintain this lofty position. Rheba's lesson learned: Success often imposes burdens at all levels.

NOT SUCCEEDING DOESN'T MEAN FAILURE

—Linda Aiken

If you don't achieve success on the first, second or third attempt, it doesn't mean you have failed. It simply means you must try again from a different angle. During an initial examination of hospital outcomes, Linda attempted to tease apart the various programs (clinical ladders, tuition benefits, shared governance, etc.) that might be contributing to better outcomes. However, no relationship could be found. After numerous attempts, it was discovered that the synergistic effect of *all* the elements produced the improved hospital outcomes. This "all-or-none" discovery led Linda and her team to study hospitals with excellent reputations, which became the outcomes evidence for developing the American Nurses Credentialing Center's Magnet Recognition Program. Never give up on a good idea—you never know where it will lead you, especially when it takes you down unexpected paths.

YOUR ACCOMPLISHMENTS DO THE TALKING

—Vernice Ferguson

Vernice created her own dreams throughout her career. She was a fighter who felt that neither race nor gender would ever get in her way. Further, "If one gets a good education and becomes excellent in what he or she does, it will be recognized and speak for itself." Vernice never makes excuses, but instead chooses to let her outcomes do the talking.

PATIENT SATISFACTION AS A MEASURE OF LEADERSHIP VALIDITY

—Margaret McClure

"If patients are unhappy with their nursing care, then they are unhappy with everything. The nurse executive's best measure for the performance of the nursing division is patient complaints—this is your validity measure."

Maggie's experience taught her that people will only take time to state an opinion if they are very happy or very angry. In 1979, when Maggie became executive director of nursing at New York University (NYU) Medical Center, she expected complaints to cross her desk. After 18 months of waiting, she approached the department of her hospital administration office and inquired about where she would find the patient complaints. She was dumbfounded when told, "We don't get complaints." At that moment, she understood how high the customer service bar was at NYU Medical Center, and it was being honored at the bedside. Maintaining this high standard of patient satisfaction was a leadership responsibility she gladly embraced. Maggie laughed when she recalled finally getting a letter of complaint. "You would have thought someone had died; we took that complaint very personally."

Lesson learned: If you want to understand the priorities of the nursing division leadership, ask to see the patient complaint log.

A Vision That Came Full Circle

—Faye Abdellah

How many nurses can remember the exact moment they made the decision to enter the nursing profession? Faye Abdellah can do just that. As a child, she was present during the crash of the Hindenburg airship on 6 May 1937. This international tragedy changed lives everywhere, including Faye's. The young girl who wanted to help others in a time of crisis went on to do just that. Faye's lifelong contribution to the profession was her vision to create an educational program for nurses that focused on disaster response. She founded the Graduate School of Nursing at Uniformed Services University of the Health Sciences in Bethesda, Maryland, USA. Her nursing students were present on 11 September 2001 when a terrorist attack on the Pentagon building in Washington, DC, occurred. From that child who looked on helplessly to the leader who founded a school to train graduate nurses in disaster response, her career had come full circle.

Can you think of a nurse on your staff or a colleague who has really made a difference to the organization or profession? Have you?

MAKE AN IMPACT

—Shirley Chater

Shirley dedicated her career to serving women and minorities. While she was at Texas Woman's University, there were programs for young girls interested in math and science, along with a program for single mothers who worked part-time jobs and held scholarships through school. The campus became home for them and their children. Another program, *De Madres a Madres* (from mother to mother), enabled pregnant Hispanic women to receive prenatal care from other Hispanic women who had gone through an educational program supervised within the School of Nursing. Shirley made a difference that would impact these women for the rest of their lives. Moments of inspiration can come when least expected and last a lifetime.

FINDING THE BALANCE

—Shirley Chater

Most leaders struggle with finding a balance among career, family, and personal time. Shirley was no different in striving to seek balance, and most of her career was a juggling act. She says, "You can think of balancing your life in two ways: One I call both/and, while the other is either/or. A lot of people think they can either go the professional route or choose to be a wife and mother. I like the both/and approach: You can have both and do both. You can enjoy a family life while leading a professional life."

LEADERSHIP TAKES TIME

—Richard Carmona

"Aligning and moving the team is like cat herding—random movement with a number of different ideas that doesn't really develop inertia or coordination. True leadership will ultimately create a team synergy. To develop as a true leader takes time, and that's the difficulty. People must be willing to subordinate their own idea of success for yours because they truly believe in you as an inspired leader. This takes years."

THE TRIPLE CROWN OF NURSING LEADERSHIP

—Gretta Styles

Gretta was an educator, researcher, administrator, and practitioner interested in developing all aspects of the profession. She devoted her career to advancing the profession in a global manner. Gretta is the only person to hold the "triple crown" of nursing leadership: president of the American Nurses Association (1986-88), president of the American Nurses Credentialing Center (1996-98), and president of the International Council of Nurses (1993-97). She fulfilled her dream.

What are your dreams? Are you taking steps to achieve them?

SEE THE WORLD FROM A DIFFERENT PERSPECTIVE

—Marla Salmon

"You can't go somewhere without leaving somewhere."

Marla's parents instilled in their children that you have to see the world to appreciate what you want and understand what you need to know. Their children all knew that when they finished high school they were expected to leave home and learn something new before they returned. Her mother believed that leaving was essential for forward progress. The easy road was to stay in the known comfort zone. Moving to new surroundings, with a new culture, might change your vision forever.

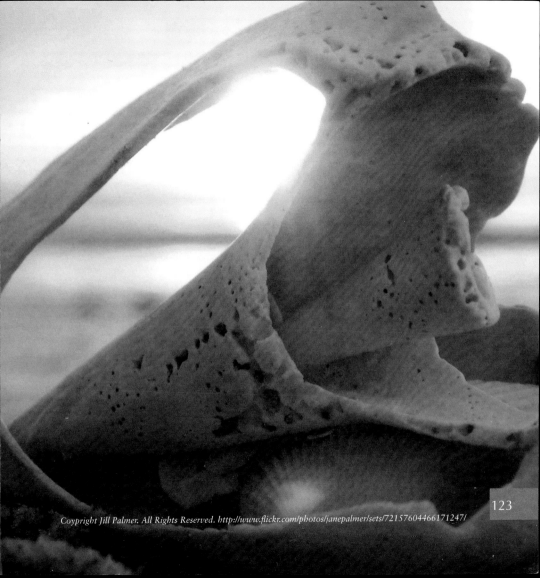

123

BOOKS PUBLISHED BY THE HONOR SOCIETY OF NURSING, SIGMA THETA TAU INTERNATIONAL

Words of Wisdom From Pivotal Nurse Leaders, Houser and Player, 2008.

Ready, Set, Go Lead! A Primer for Emerging Health Care Leaders, Dickenson-Hazard, 2008.

Tales From The Pager Chronicles, Rancour, 2008.

The Nurse's Etiquette Advantage, Pagana, 2008.

NURSE: A World of Care, Jaret, 2008. Published by Emory University and distributed by the Honor Society of Nursing, Sigma Theta Tau International.

Johns Hopkins Nursing Evidence-Based Practice Model and Guidelines, Newhouse, Dearholt, Poe, Pugh, and White, 2007.

Nursing Without Borders: Values, Wisdom, Success Markers, Weinstein and Brooks, 2007.

Synergy: The Unique Relationship Between Nurses and Patients, Curley, 2007.

Conversations With Leaders: Frank Talk From Nurses (and Others) on the Front Lines of Leadership, Hansen-Turton, Sherman, and Ferguson, 2007.

Pivotal Moments in Nursing: Leaders Who Changed the Path of a Profession, Houser and Player, 2004 (Volume I) and 2007 (Volume II).

Shared Legacy, Shared Vision: The W.K. Kellogg Foundation and the Nursing Profession, Lynaugh, Smith, Grace, Sena, de Villalobos, and Hlalele, 2007.

Daily Miracles: Stories and Practices of Humanity and Excellence in Health Care, Briskin and Boller, 2006.

A Daybook for Nurse Leaders and Mentors. Sigma Theta Tau International, 2006.

When Parents Say No: Religious and Cultural Influences on Pediatric Healthcare Treatment, Linnard-Palmer, 2006.

Healthy Places, Healthy People: A Handbook for Culturally Competent Community Nursing Practice, Dreher, Shapiro, and Asselin, 2006.

The HeART of Nursing: Expressions of Creative Art in Nursing, Second Edition, Wendler, 2005.

Technological Competency as Caring in Nursing, Locsin, 2005.

Making a Difference: Stories from the Point of Care, Volume I, Hudacek, 2005.

A Daybook for Nurses: Making a Difference Each Day, Hudacek, 2004.

Making a Difference: Stories from the Point of Care, Volume II, Hudacek, 2004.

Ordinary People, Extraordinary Lives: The Stories of Nurses, Smeltzer and Vlasses, 2003.

For more information and to order these books from the Honor Society of Nursing, Sigma Theta Tau International, visit the society's Web site at www.nursingsociety.org/publications, or go to www.nursingknowledge.org/stti/books, the Web site of Nursing Knowledge International, the honor society's sales and distribution division, or call 1.888.NKI.4.YOU (U.S. and Canada) or +1.317.634.8171 (Outside U.S. and Canada).